LEVEL UP YOUR MEDICAL SPA

#1 Technician Resource Consults to Increased Sales

ANGELA JAWORSKI

COPYRIGHT PAGE

ISBN: 979-8-9872110-6-9

CONTENTS

Introduction   v

1. Anatomy associated with Body Contouring   1
   (bonus; details on Cellulite and stretch marks)

2. Factors that affect the body and client results
   or lack of   19
   (bonus; details on belly shape meanings)

3. Types of nonsurgical technologies and how
   they affect the body   25
   (know your competitor)

4. Client consult and communication; obtain and
   retain your clients   47

5. Client consult and communication; obtain and
   retain your clients   69

6. Botox, fillers, and how they compare to non-
   surgical treatments   73

7. Marketing YOUR business; with/without
   clients, lipo aftercare, mommy pouch care   79

8. pening a medical spa; staffing details,
   insurance, licensing, treatment room and
   consumables list, equipment recommendations   113

   Workbook Questions   123

   Glossary   129

9. Generic Face/Body Consent Form   143

   Get Your Questions Answered   147

INTRODUCTION

Hello and thank you for purchasing my book. I am Angela Jaworski, a licensed esthetician, certified equipment trainer, and consultant. I want to share with you why I created this book and joined the industry. It started when I went from 240 lbs. to 155 lbs.

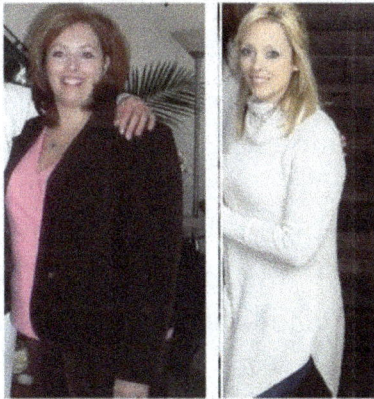

In 2005, what felt like a mortifying moment allowed me to see what I had become, 240 lbs., and realizing my self-worth was connected to being overweight. The next day I started down a road, unknowingly, to nowhere; I fell for fad diets and took prescription weight loss pills that helped to lose 40 lbs. but harmed my nutrition, my vision and my hair.

After a relationship loss and some self-reflection, I realized I'd never given myself the time, energy and accountability I deserved. So I left the diets and prescription pills behind. Instead, I made changes that included 30 minutes of daily activity, reviewing my food intake to remove poor choices and improve the quality of my calories. As a result, in one year, I went from 220 lbs. to 160 lbs. No diet pills, just truly giving to myself.

After all that and to still have so much excess skin. I learned that I didn't know the value of taking care of my skin during my weight loss. Unfamiliar with non-surgical options, I ended up with two surgeries. The first one was to remove the excess skin and repair an unknown hernia. When the results weren't as expected or healing properly, I was demeaned by my surgeon and told the results were my fault. The second surgery happened four years later to address an unhealed belly button, improperly attached skin, and remove 3 lbs. of skin left from the prior surgery. The surgical and emotional pain I went through is hard to express, but it changed my life. From this journey, my passion ignited. As I became aware of the non-surgical world, I realized how this method could have possibly saved me from two surgeries and to understand that quality of life while making changes and improvements does matter. So I dove into researching every technology available in the market, how they work, who can provide them, and how I could change my entire career to help others avoid what I went through.

Taking my professional background into review in my business degree and education in massage therapy, where I studied anatomy and physiology, I knew that the best approach for me to help others was to become an Esthetician. I put myself through school, took on an apprenticeship, passed the state licensing, and worked with a Med Spa in Ann Arbor, Michigan; as if that wasn't enough, I also trained with the manufacturer on all the equipment we used and became a nationally certified trainer for that manufacturer. With my growing thirst for knowledge, I joined others within the aesthetic community to discuss client results and new techniques to maximize results safely and continuously learn how to best serve my clients. This entire journey resulted in owning my own spa and later selling it to move from Michigan to Colorado, assisting spas in successfully opening, and consulting other professionals on how to do what I do.

I went from working in corporate America counting down the hours to loving the work I do every day, excited to hear the life journey of my next client and how I can help. As well as, create a positive environment for my clients to achieve results in a JUDGMENT-FREE ZONE. We all have our own path and it's no one's place to judge where we've been, especially if we are working towards our better selves. Inspiring others to take a more natural approach to body contouring, so they can feel their most natural, beautiful self is why I do what I do, and created this book for the non-surgical industry. Thank you again for taking the time to read this book and understanding my "Why." Why I love what I do, why I put this book together, and I hope it helps increase your love for this industry.

In this book, you will review the basic anatomy to understand how non-surgical options work with the body, factors affecting the body and results, types of technologies (as there are more machine names and manufacturers than types of technology), consultations, how to communicate with clients, photos to help understand the information and bonus material about Cellulite, insight into body shapes, starting a medical spa, how to breakdown treatment pricing, and marketing your business if you are starting with or without a client base.

Also, in the back, is a list of questions to help you retain the complex information supplied in this book. Should you have comments or questions or would like

my equipment training and consultation services, you can email me at contournetics@gmail.com.

1

ANATOMY ASSOCIATED WITH BODY CONTOURING

(bonus; details on Cellulite and stretch marks)

I'M SO excited to share this information. Let's get started! Obtaining successful results includes knowing the anatomy affected by non-surgical body contouring treatments and some bonus details on Cellulite and stretch marks.

If you have yet to study anatomy and physiology, the review in this chapter will be simple, streamlined and extremely helpful in understanding how treatments work. If you are knowledgeable in anatomy and physiology, then it will be an excellent refresher in a more focused presentation. In most cases, our bodies start with everything they need to function. In a beautifully complex system, our bodies are self-powered and begin with the heartbeat, pushing all the blood and fluids through an intricate maze that fuels a diverse group of organs and filter the difference between nutrients and waste.

Within this robust system, non-surgical body contouring affects fat cells, the lymphatic system, and our skin-the largest organ of the body, focused more on the collagen and elastin within the skin. Photo from: "image: Dreamstime.-com". Contributing image asset from Dreamstime.com

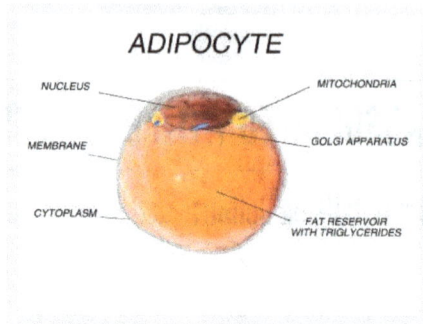

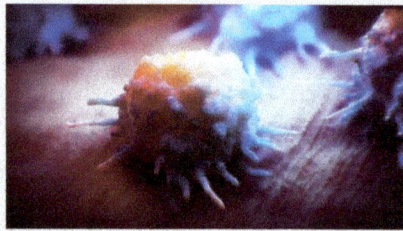

We are starting with a review of the fat cell and where it is located. First, we must understand the purpose of fat cells and how they work in the body. Your body starts with all the healthy fat cells it needs to function roughly by age seven. Then the types of meals and beverages we consume turn into fat that is designed to be stored and burned for energy as needed. Finally, the fats that are not naturally in our bodies are labeled toxins.

To further explain toxins, it helps to know they are considered carbohydrates, sugar, bad fatty

foods, and alcohol. Another contributing factor to fat cells is high cortisol levels; they can increase fat storage, typically found around the abdomen. When we become active, we exert this stored energy, and the toxins break away from the healthy fat cell and enter the bloodstream. Eventually, the toxins break down enough to exit the body in any way possible; urine, bowel movements, ear wax, sweat and even through your breath. When we consume more toxins than exerting energy, the toxins continue to accumulate, backing up and waiting for the liver to process. Over time the new consumed toxins are flushed out first and the older toxins become harder to discard. Causing the fat cells to enlarge, expanding the skin and creating the body shape we do not want.

There are two locations where our fat cells reside, so they have different names, visceral fat (which is around the organs under the muscle. The second name is subcutaneous fat (affected by surgical and non-surgical options), located between the muscle and skin layers.

Photo from: "image: Dreamstime.com". Contributing image asset from Dreamstime.com

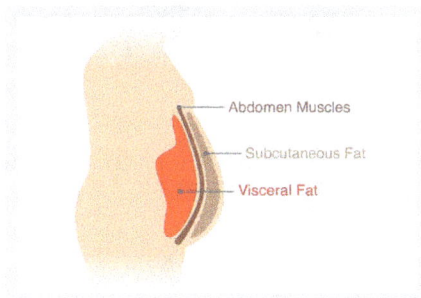

We will go over visceral fat first. It is located around the organs and underneath the bone and muscle structure. When toxins enter the body, they attach to the fat cells

starting with the visceral fat. These cells have many functions, such as

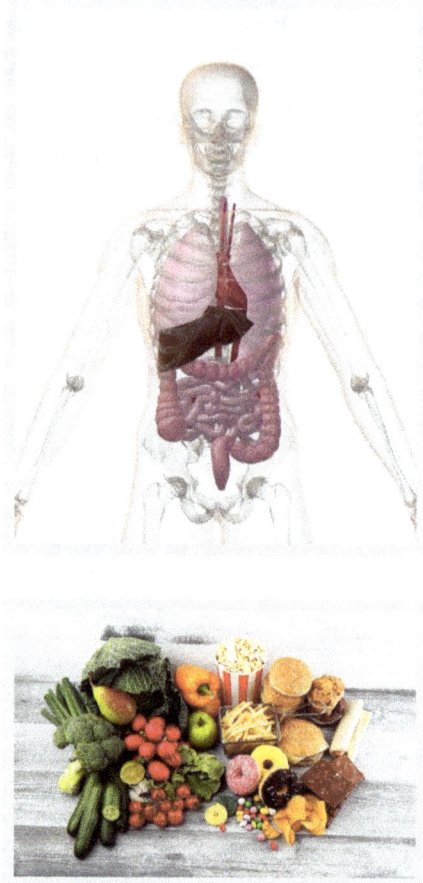

Photo from: "image: Dreamstime.com". Contributing image asset from Dreamstime.com

protecting the organs, collecting vital nutrients, and balancing cholesterol and blood pressure. The visceral fat is limited in expanding due to the bone structure and the surrounding muscle. If we do not initiate proper physical activity, our bodies will not burn what is supposed to be temporarily stored fat. The toxins will accumulate and begin to attach to the subcutaneous fat once there is no more room in the visceral fat area.

When you initiate physical activity, the body will eliminate the toxins from the visceral fat first. This is why we do not see the shape of our body change over the first 30 days. Additionally, one reason why a balanced diet and active life-style matters is because visceral fat is the closest to the liver and creates a higher risk to the health of the body.

Subcutaneous fat is located between the muscle and skin to protect the bone and muscle upon impact and is a pathway for nerves and blood vessels. Too much in this area stretches the skin and the structural resources to support skin and most importantly increases health risks. See the enlarged photo below to show how excess subcutaneous fat stretches the skin's structure.

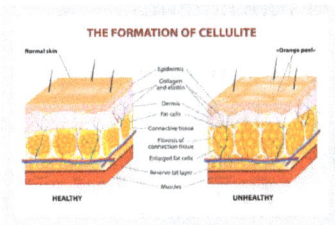

THE FORMATION OF CELLULITE

The subcutaneous fat is less risky and the last to leave the body. Although this fact is why someone chooses a non-surgical option to remove subcutaneous fat, the client must work on a balanced diet and be active to help eliminate the excess toxins in the visceral fat. It cannot be destroyed by surgical or non-surgical options (because of its location.)

Now that we have covered the types of fat, we will review the lymphatic system.

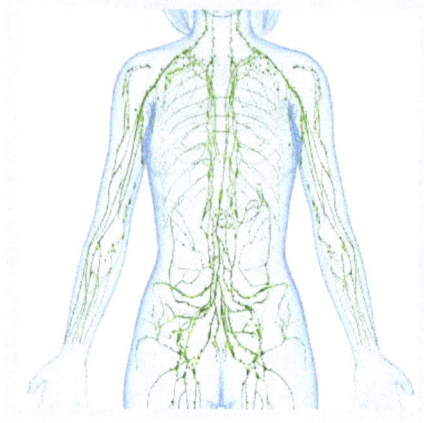

The lymphatic system has three functions, and for this book, we will focus on how it works on just removing toxins. A simplified explanation is when the body becomes active, the lymphatic fluid moves through the body, collecting excess fluids and toxins, moving them out through the bloodstream and exiting the body, most typically into the small intestine and out through secretion (aka a bowel movement.)

For the body to create the pumping action needed to move the lymph fluid through the body, the body needs to be intentionally moving, or a simple lymphatic massage can provide assistance. With all of this in mind, we should remember how the melting process affects the body. Refer back to the description of fat cells; when the toxins break away entering the lymphatic and the bloodstream, potentially affecting a client's blood pressure, triglycerides, and cholesterol levels. Therefore, it is vital to receive and thoroughly review the client's intake form.

Also, the combination of the breakdown of fat and the lymph system is why when clients ask how they see results immediately. The non-surgical technology breaks away the toxins from the healthy fat cell in the subcutaneous layers and disperses them into the lymphatic system and bloodstream to exit the body. This disbursement is why you no longer see the fat volume in the treatment area. The client being active after treatment and drinking plenty of water will help support flushing their system. Here is a great example I give my clients. Imagine a stack of ice cubes in a glass. Notice how quick it will fill the glass to the top. When the ice melts it takes up less space in the glass because it is dispersed differently. In this case of non-surgical treatments the fat cell is destroyed (melted) and pushed to the lymphatic to be flushed out.

Let's move on to the skin. The skin consists of three main layers: epidermis, dermis and hypodermis.

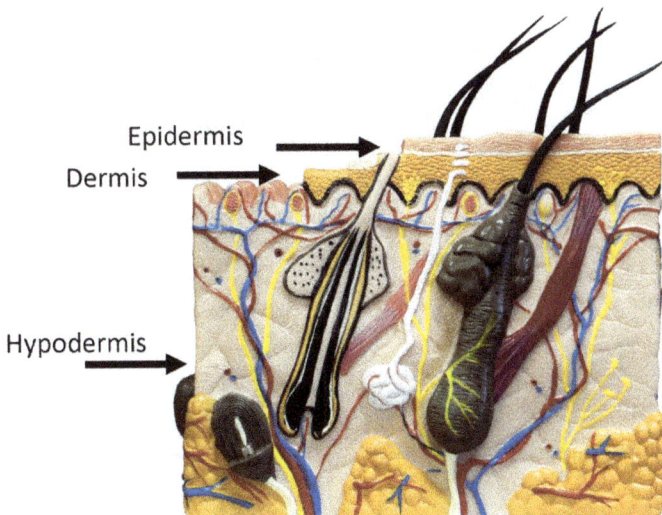

Most of you probably remember the epidermis is the outer-most layer providing a waterproof barrier and our skin tone. The dermis holds the sweat glands, hair follicles, and connective tissue, while the hypodermis contains the connective tissue and fat cells.

In the non-surgical world, the melting fat and skin tight-ening procedures affect the epidermis and hypodermis layers. They provide the structure and shape for the bodies we see in the mirror. As we age or after childbirth, we know our collagen and elastin production decreases and is a vital part of helping the structure in the dermis layer of our skin.

When we gain or lose weight, the structural support system designed within our skin gets compromised; hence the appearance of stretch marks.

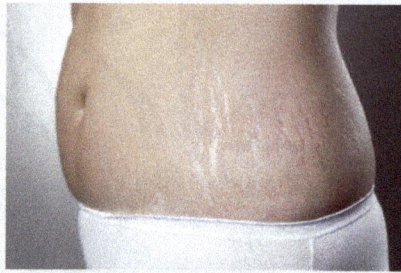

However, depending on an individual's age, diet, and genet-ics, some may never experience stretch marks. Stretch marks are still an anomaly to some, and in the beginning, I searched high and low for a simple explanation for why eliminating them can be so challenging. From a great discus-sion with the head of plastic surgery at Beaumont hospital, the primary explanation for stretch marks is briefly described as tears through the layers of the skin, similar to what happens with a scar. This compromise of the skin empties the functioning cellular structure as almost a void. The best we can do as providers is to stimulate the good skin around the stretch marks to maximize the support along the sides of the stretch mark to rebuild the collagen and elastin, which improves the support structure and minimizes the appearance of the stretch marks.

When the skin becomes compromised, we begin to see skin like in the photo provided.

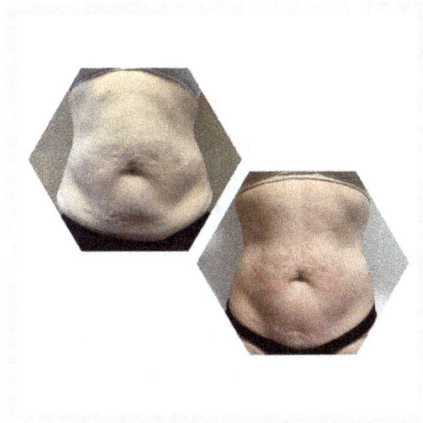

In this photo, you see skin that has undergone surgery, stretch marks, and weight loss. Your role as a provider or technician is to help determine how to achieve the client's goals, and decide whether they need skin tightening, fat melting or both.

Sometimes the difference between loose skin and stubborn fat is pronounced, such as the skin appearing wrinkled, having folds, or a crepey appearance. The less obvious can be, for example the less obvious can be after a client has had a large weight loss, but not yet reached their optimal healthy weight goal. This typically is the area around the abdomen.

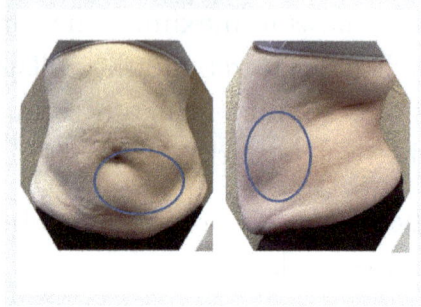

Referring to the photo as I continue, when looking around the belly button, it is most likely more fat than loose skin if it is smooth and uniform in appearance. If the area is rippled or droopy, it is most likely loose skin with some fat underneath.

A little bonus material, we will review the details of one big question in the contouring industry among providers and clients. To some, an unpleasant word, Cellulite. Can you get rid of the Cellulite?

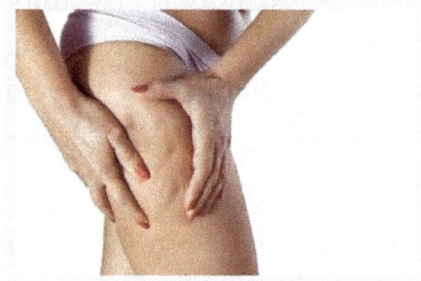

While the exact cause of Cellulite is unknown, and how to permanently eliminate it is yet to be solved, we can review what makes up Cellulite and how we may be able to diminish and potentially keep it at bay.

There are three types of Cellulite, several factors that affect it, and stages of lymphatic obstructions contributing to Cellulite appearance. The three types of Cellulite, Aqueous (Grade 1), Adipose (Grade 2), and Fibrous (Grade 3):

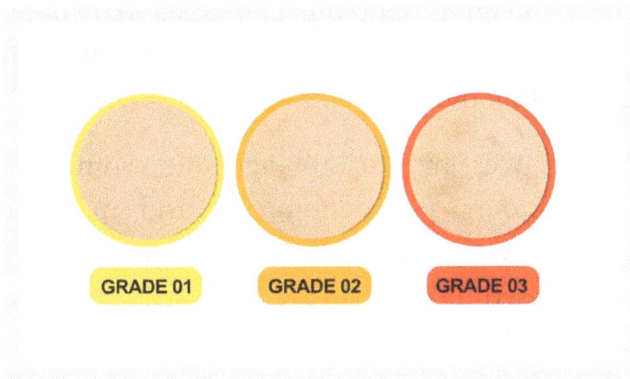

GRADE 01   GRADE 02   GRADE 03

A-qwe-ous Cellulite happens with poor circulation and water retention. As a result the skin is similar to an orange peel, tight and not soft.

Adipose Cellulite is the easiest to eliminate as it is due to excess fat (or also described in the treatment room as excess volume) in the area causing structural stress, you can pinch the skin to see it, and it does not hurt.

Fibrous Cellulite happens when the collagen fibers around the fat cells harden. The Cellulite is very visible and, when pinched, can be painful to the touch. This type of Cellulite is the most difficult to eliminate.

A good site to review more information is in the link provided   https://www.cellublue.com/blog/en/your-Cellulite-type/

In the photo below you can see more clearly, under the dermis layer, the strained structure and excess fat contributing to the Cellulite.

The factors affecting Cellulite include; Hormones, Age, Genetic Factors, Skin Structure, Fat distribution, Diet, Smoking, and Inactivity. We will review these now.

Hormone changes at various ages in women, such as puberty, pregnancy, perimenopause, and menopause, all play a factor in weight gain and loss. In addition, the pressure of increased fat on our connective tissue structure increases the visibility of Cellulite.

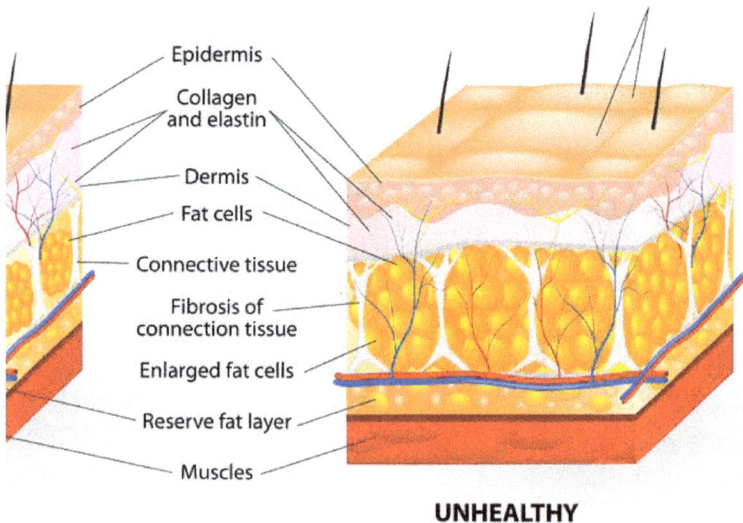

Epidermis

Collagen and elastin

Dermis

Fat cells

Connective tissue

Fibrosis of connection tissue

Enlarged fat cells

Reserve fat layer

Muscles

UNHEALTHY

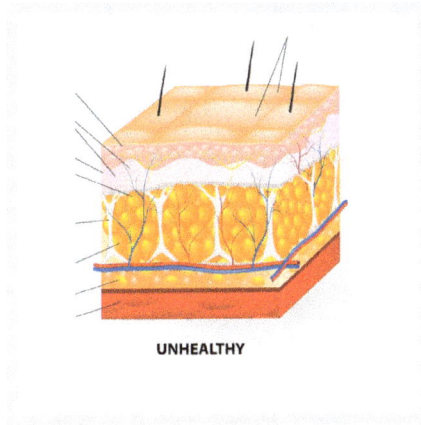

UNHEALTHY

Aging affects the cellular structure within our body to the point where the ability to maintain the structure is decreased. However, keeping a balanced diet and active life-style does contribute to minimizing the effects.

Regarding genetics, they have found in women that the connective tissues and fat cells are structured vertically, while they are a criss-cross in men. As shown in the photo.

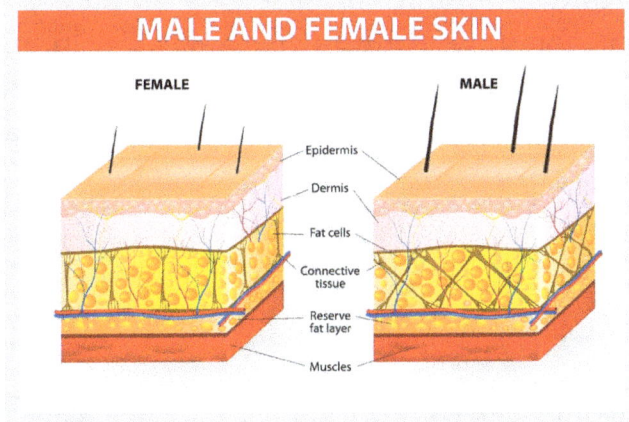

MALE AND FEMALE SKIN

FEMALE   MALE

Epidermis

Dermis

Fat cells

Connective tissue

Reserve fat layer

Muscles

The more supportive structure in men is why they seem to have less visible Cellulite. Additionally, individual genetics can cause the developing connective tissue to have limitations in its ability to maintain its structure. Some may inherit genes that have a tighter fibrous band (connective tissue) than others. The lack of flexibility makes any level of fat build-up visible.

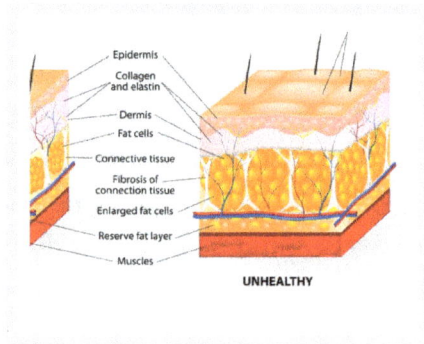

Epidermis
Collagen and elastin
Dermis
Fat cells
Connective tissue
Fibrosis of connection tissue
Enlarged fat cells
Reserve fat layer
Muscles

UNHEALTHY

Treatments for Cellulite at any level are currently not permanent. However, maintaining a balanced diet, staying active, providing healthy collagen support, and, if desired, occasional non-surgical treatments will all help and work together to keep Cellulite at bay. Researchers and scientists are still working on providing a more permanent solution.

A client, who smokes, can potentially be a significant factor for Cellulite, as well as affecting their body overall. Smoking actually constricts the blood vessels lowering the oxygen flow to the dermis layer of the skin. With the skin being the body's largest organ of the body it is helpful to remind clients the importance of taking care of their skin. In addition, the lack of oxygen decreases the function of the circulatory system and the flow of the lymphatic system, making it challenging to achieve optimal non-surgical results.

Continuing with factors affecting Cellulite, inactivity slows down collagen and elastin production and affects the entire function of the body as well as your overall health. Activity is vital as it initiates the heart's pumping action, creating a chain reaction within the entire body.

In keeping with non-surgical treatment purposes, the lymphatic system is activated by the heart's pumping action so it can flush out the toxins that have broken off the healthy fat cell. A great example I share is "Imaging cooking your family an entire breakfast in one skillet. Afterward, you go to clean it. You put in the soap and start to scrub, and someone yells to you, "Oh my gosh, you have to see this!" You put the pan upside-down to look at, and by the time you come back, you see some of the soap has drained out. But is it clean? No. You would think to yourself if you had only taken action to turn on the faucet and run the water over the pan, you would not have to scrub again to finish cleaning it. Your turning on the faucet is the same as the client being physically active. The water running to clean the pan is the value of drinking enough water to support flushing the body of toxins. This analogy seems to connect and be the most understandable example, with my clients.

Wrapping up understanding Cellulite, we will review lymphatic blockages. Depending on which medical source you refer to, some say there are four blockages and others say five. We will go ahead and cover all five stages:

- **Stage 1 Cellulite** is only visible when forced; otherwise, it is unseen.
- **Stage 2 Cellulite** is slightly visible while standing or pinching the skin, such as the legs crossing.
- **Stage 3 Cellulite** is visible while standing; no force is needed the skin is soft and moveable.
- **Stage 4 Cellulite** is visible while standing. Area is hardened.
- **Stage 5 Cellulite** is visible while standing and the skin is tight and hard.

Let's dive more into these stages.

Stage one is the beginning phase of Cellulite that is affected by decreased lymphatic flow, blood flow, and or fluid retention. This stage is treatable by non-surgical body contouring.

Stage two is the continued decrease in lymphatic flow, blood flow, and increase in fluid retention, and it is also treatable by non-surgical body contouring.

Stage three, while all of stage one and two indicators apply, the fat layer under the skin has also increased and is starting to push against the skin. However, the skin is still soft, moveable, and treatable by non-surgical options. As you advance in stages, the increase in the number of treatments will be necessary to get results, and then the client will go into maintenance mode.

Stage 4 Cellulite is typically when a client's lymphatic flow has become somewhat dormant; genetics may also be a factor. The increased slowing down of the lymphatic system and blood flow starts to block fat from being flushed from the body, decreasing the normal oxygen flow to the overall area. The lack of fluidity starts to harden this area. Again, non-Surgical treatments are possible, however complete elimination of Cellulite is going to be a lot more difficult to achieve.

In Stage 5 the indicators show the blockages are more significant within the lymphatic system, the flow of blood and genetics are a higher possibility that non-surgical treatments will help along with some suggested lymphatic massage (note: this is a great recommendation at all stages in my experience.) Yet stage 5 is the most difficult to achieve optimal results, where elimination may not be achieved, and diminishing the appearance will be your most likely result.

That completes our chapter on Cellulite, what causes Cellulite, and how we, as providers and technicians can affect the stages of Cellulite.

DIFFERENT STAGES OF CELLULITE

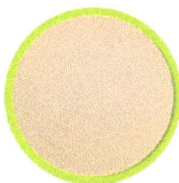

GRADE 00	GRADE 01	GRADE 02	GRADE 03
No dimpling when pressure is applied	Dimpling when pressure is applied	Dimpling is visible when standing, but not when lying down	Dimpling while both when standing and lying down

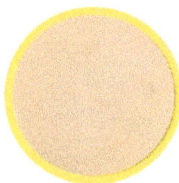

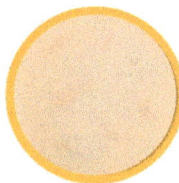

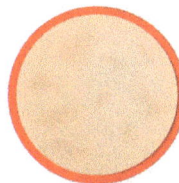

2

FACTORS THAT AFFECT THE BODY AND CLIENT RESULTS OR LACK OF

(bonus; details on belly shape meanings)

WHILE OUR TRAINING shows providers how to apply the treatments, we should understand what factors contribute to a client's current body size, shape and results; this includes food, activity, water intake, hormones, and skin responsiveness. So let's review all of these in detail.

We'll get started with food and its effects on the body this includes; light food allergies and excessive eating.

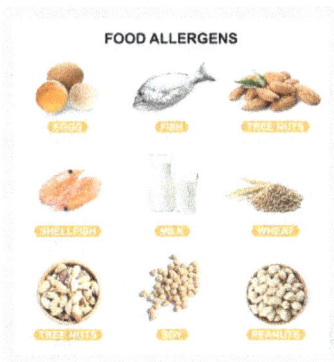

FOOD ALLERGENS

Light food allergies can cause the body not to process food correctly. An example we will go with is sugar. When the body has difficulty processing the sugars consumed the skin fibers will retain excess glucose. This is what we call glycation. It shows up as deep wrinkles around the mouth, making it harder for the skin to respond to tighten treatments.

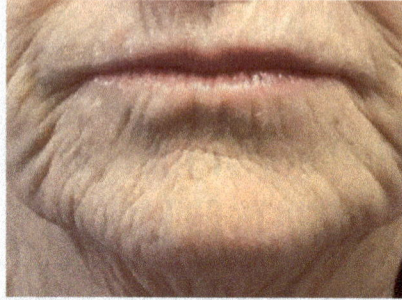

A food allergy can also create internal inflammation, water retention, and or potential clogging of the digestive tract that may not allow a complete healthy clearing of the digestive system.

Excessive eating, be it a variety of bad food or too much of one type of food, this imbalance of proper nutrition does not allow the body enough time to burn the energy stored, especially if it is constantly fed too much. This lifestyle is why many health experts state a balance of diet and daily activity are needed.

The level of physical activity and suitable activity is essential to non-surgical treatments. Cardio is the most recommended and valuable for non-surgical treatments. Types of Cardio workouts can include; fast walking, hiking, dancing, and kickboxing. These are all examples of what you can suggest to your clients for at least three days following treatment, no less than 15 minutes a day; however, 20 to 30 minutes is most effective. Cardio activity, as mentioned in chapter one, stimulates the lymphatic system to flush the broken-down fat out of the body. You can review chapter one again regarding how the lymphatic system works.

When talking about activity, your Clients will ask about weight lifting to increase muscle tone. This type of activity is not preferred right after treatment. Building muscle does stimulate the lymphatic; however, the body focuses more on building muscle mass and bone density than it does on flushing the broken-down fat out of the body. Clients can resume muscle building typically no sooner than three days after each treatment.

The level of water intake also plays a vital role in treatment success. The body uses water to hydrate and support the organs, including the skin. Water is a valuable contributing factor for non-surgical treatments and flushing out toxins. You need to emphasize the importance of water with your clients. A relatable analogy I mentioned in chapter one, is washing the skillet. Just a refresher, we'll go over it again;

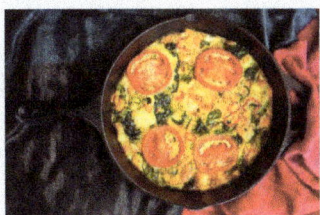

You've cooked your meal in one pan and after dinner, you go to the sink, apply the soap, and start scrubbing. A family member says you have to come quick, don't miss this, so you tip the pan upside down and run over. An hour or so goes by, and you remember you never finished cleaning that pan. Flipping it over, you see that some food residue has drained off; however, it is not completely clean. Had you turned on the water entirely to rinse the pan out before you left earlier, it would have eliminated the entire food residue. This great example is why drinking enough water is vital in maximizing treatments.

Some clients state they have issues drinking water; this could be due to an acid reflux issue or something to mention to their doctor or naturopath. In the meantime, here are some tips to help clients increase their water intake;

1. Every time they look at the clock, they drink water.
2. At each meal, ensure that two cups (or 16oz) of water are consumed.
3. Start small with ¼ cup of water every waking hour, then increase the hourly water intake each day or week.

Hormone imbalance is another contributing factor that can be caused by stress levels, medications like birth control, post pregnancy, and menopause. Having your hormones out of balance can affect a client's weight, ability to lose weight, cause inflammation, and excessive water retention.

This type of complication reduces the effectiveness of non-surgical treatments. If your spa location cannot test for these concerns, having a list of external referral resources has proven to be a bonus for client retention and word-of-mouth referrals. I call this the miracle on 34th street approach. We will review more referral resources in the marketing chapter.

Some topics that affect the body, its shape, and how the skin responds include a client's genetics such as being more prone to stretch marks. Extreme environmental factors include climate, elevation, diet, and air pollution. Additionally, age plays a role in further explaining skin response in aging after age 35 or after having children. Because the collagen and elastin production decreases, making it more difficult for the skin to tighten on its own; this is where non-surgical options that tighten are most beneficial.

3

TYPES OF NONSURGICAL TECHNOLOGIES AND HOW THEY AFFECT THE BODY

(know your competitor)

THE NON-SURGICAL FACE and body contouring industry has so many machines on the market that it is challenging to keep up with what is the best, especially when combining technologies on these machines. To help simplify, it helps to understand the technology. So what technologies are available, the basics of how they work, and what is the general treatment cost?

In general, there are six types of technology in the non-surgical contouring industry; cryo lipolysis, laser lipolysis, radio frequency, combined infrared with red light therapy, electromagnetic muscle stimulation, and ultrasound cavitation. Finally, this section will discuss how to describe to your clients the difference between surgical and non-surgical.

CRYO LIPOLYSIS (CRYO-LIPO-LYSIS)

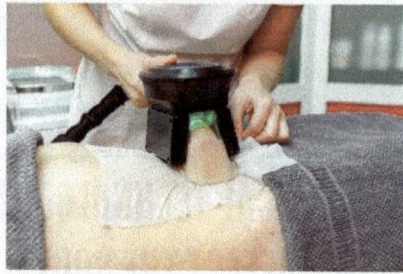

also known as "the freezing of fat." This treatment works through the anatomy because it affects the skin first, then the tissue and lastly, the fat cells, freezing each layer. This treatment has a special protective wet cloth placed over the treatment area to protect the skin, as shown in the photo above. Next, the technician places the handle onto the client's treatment area. The handle has two functions, suction and freezing. First, the suction settings create a vacuum sensation that pulls the skin into the handle. When that is complete, the cryo (freezing) feature slowly drops the temperature, where the fat cell is then frozen, and the toxins cannot keep their attachment to the healthy fat cell, and break away. After the technician turns on the machine to start the treatment, they typically leave the room and return periodically to check on the client until the treatment is complete, as it automatically turns off. Your trainer will state not to allow the client to remove the applicator themselves as post-care is required immediately after so that the client does not injure themselves or damage the machine.

Post-care includes massaging the treatment area until the topical feel of the skin is closer to the temperature of the surrounding skin. The freezing and thawing during treatment will give the client a level of pain and or discomfort, which is why some professionals provide pain medication.

The number of treatments will depend on how much fat the client wants to eliminate. Small stubborn areas potentially one treatment, if looking to lose 1 to 2 inches. Clients requiring more than a couple of inches eliminated will require multiple sessions and possibly more than one treatment area. The photo provided shows one handle and one treatment area.

How often the client can receive treatment is between 6-8 weeks to ensure the skin's safety. Treating too soon presents a possibility of over-freezing the treatment area, which could cause irreversible damage to the skin or underlying tissue. Post-care for clients is very important. If the area is not massaged long enough bringing the skin temperature back to normal, the area could harden. This is called paradoxical adipose hyperplasia ((abnormal)(fat) and unusual increase in structure). I would also like to mention that studies show there are a small number of cases where clients have a reverse effect from freezing treatments. This effect causes an increase in fat cells as the body tries to protect itself.

Regarding how effective it is on skin tightening, this treatment relies on the clients' skin to naturally retract and tighten on its own. Although no current studies are proving that this treatment will induce skin tightening, it does potentially present dermal thickening giving the appearance of tightened skin.

Treatment areas for this technology include the following areas; the chin, arms, stomach, flanks, buttocks and thighs. Treatment costs range from $600 to $800 per applicator in a treatment area for one session. When using this technology, you want to understand how the machine works, and ensuring you receive proper training from the manufacturer is extremely important. Operating this machine with little information creates a risk to the client and your business. Please seek out all instructions from your manufacturer and sales representative. If they do not provide proper thorough training, I encourage you to seek a representative that trains specifically on your machine; it will be worth your time and money as client safety should be your number one priority.

Some providers and clients may need clarification on the different cryo technologies if a client mentions they have heard of "cryotherapy" reducing fat. Cryotherapy has a different effect on the body than Cryo lipolysis.

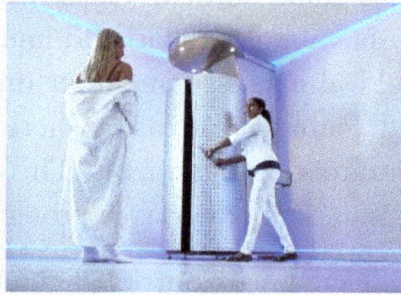

Cryotherapy offers muscular recovery and reduced inflammation after intense physical activity. To reduce fat cells, studies show it would require exposure for 2 hours, six days a week to reduce body fat by 2%, which is very different from cryo lipolysis. Cryotherapy machines include ice baths and the new trend of a stand-up booth called freezing chambers using nitrogen. This technology would not be a time-efficient or cost-effect option for clients once explained to them.

Laser lipolysis: Laser Lipolysis can be performed surgically and non-surgically for this book we are only discussing non-surgical options.

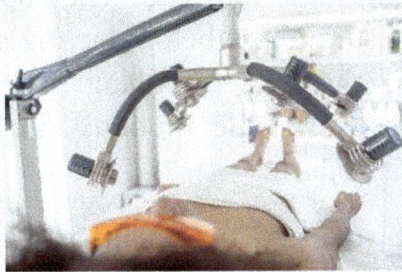

Laser Lipolysis affects the treatment area by heating the skin, tissue, and last, the fat. Depending on the chosen model, the laser energy goes through an applicator handle placed on the body or hovering over the body. The laser energy is designed to generate a level of heat projected into the treatment area for a limited time to diminish damage to the skin and tissue. The applicator used for this treatment does vary depending on the manufacturer. There is the type of applicator that hovers over the body, and the technician will cover the surrounding areas that are not being treated. Many have the other applicator, which is sometimes described as looking like a brick due to its shape. The technician will determine how many applicators are needed to cover the treatment area. They are applied flat onto the body and fastened together like a belt around the treatment area. Once the treatment is turned on, the technician usually leaves the room and periodically checks on the client until the treatment is complete. For the client's safety, do not let a client remove the applicators. With proper settings directed by the manufacturer and trainer, when the laser energy is turned on throughout the treatment, the laser energy generates a level of heat to melt the fat which also affects the skin and tissue temperature. Some applicators have a built-in cooling system that will turn on during treatment to ensure the skin and tissue does not become overheated. Please be sure to ask before buying if their machine has the built-in cooling system, asking "where is it located" and "how does it work." Be cautious using a system that does not have this built-in.

The Number of standard treatments will depend on how much fat is in the treatment area. Small stubborn areas, for example, wanting to lose 1 or 2 inches in the waist, can achieve desired results in 1-2 treatments. Typically a client with more inches to lose will need additional treatments. The average client will come in for 6-8 sessions. The minimum time between sessions is four weeks. This protocol ensures the skin's safety and does not overheat the treatment area too often. As with all treatments to the body, be sure to ask the manufacturer for post-care instructions if they are not provided. With any heat-generated treatments, the client should try not to overexert themselves with exercise to the point that their body temperature increases causing sweating or to immerse their bodies in such places as hot showers, baths, and hot tubs. The possibility of skin tightening with laser technology, there is potential to tighten as the heat will create a disturbance in the skin; however, it mainly relies on your skin to do most of the work. This is not ideal for clients who are looking to eliminate a lot of fat. In the treatment room we refer to fat as volume to ensure awareness of any sensitivity the client may have to the technical word "fat."

Treatment areas can include the chin, arms, upper, lower back, stomach, flanks, buttock, and thighs.

The cost per treatment depends on the machine and the size of the applicators. For example, the hovering applicator can range from $1500 to 3000. On the other hand, the brick applicators can range from $200 to $350 per brick-shaped applicator. For a treatment example, a lower stomach can range from 2 to 4 bricks, pricing one treatment at $400 to 1400.

Radio Frequency lipolysis: Radiofrequency, or RF for short, affects the treatment area by heating the skin, then the tissue and last breaks down the fat.

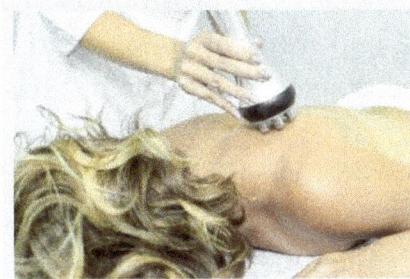

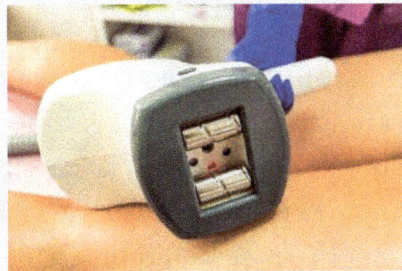

Most applicators are designed to keep the radio frequency source one centimeter away from the skin. Please be aware if your radio frequency applicator has a skin temperature monitor or comes with one separately. It is imperative to monitor the skin's temperature to ensure no damage is done through overheating. Radiofrequency is adjusted higher or lower based on the treatment areas. When treating the body, the frequency will be higher so that the heat generated will reach the subcutaneous fat layer. Resulting in the skin and tissue heating up as well; this is where the temperature monitor is helpful. Should a client not need fat reduction, this technology is the number one way to stimulate skin tightening, using lower frequency setting. The RF will disrupt the skin layers to stimulate collagen, improve elastin, and give a more rejuvenated skin appearance. You would need to refer to your manufacturer and trainer for proper settings. Radiofrequency can provide treatments to the face, chin, neck, arms, and trunk of the body, thighs, and calves, depending on the range of the machine you purchase. The number of treatments can vary depending on client goals; the average is 6 to 8. My professional opinion is that this technology works best for skin tightening over melting fat. As a result, combining this technology with ultrasound cavitation has been very effective. We will review ultrasound cavitation a little later.

The cost per treatment does depend on your applicator. An example is the known machine TruSculpt, which per a google search; you will find that it can average around $2000 to cover the abdomen and flanks, whereas two treatments for the chin with jowls would be about $1000 total.

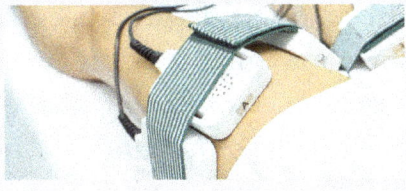

Other RF machines that provide skin tightening can average $200 for the size of the abdomen area per treatment.

Infrared and Red Light Therapy: Infrared technology does heat the skin, then the tissue, and last the fat, while red light therapy helps accelerate the metabolism, which minimizes the heat on the skin. Not all machines combine the two. The infrared energy heat penetrates the skin to 1.5 inches breaking down the toxins from the fat cell.

- Epidermis (outer skin) Dermis (glands, hair & connective tissue)
- Hypodermis (connective tissue & fat cells)

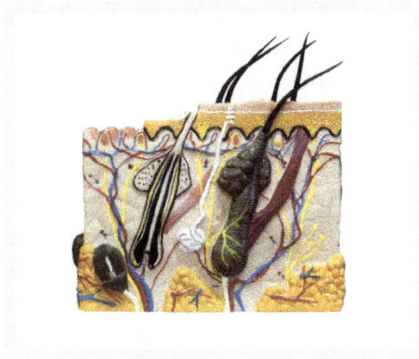

Red light is a newer technology known as photobiomodulation. It reaches the dermal layer to stimulate cellular energy, increasing metabolism and breaking down the toxins from the fat cell. This technology has also been known to reduce inflammation and autoimmune activity in the thyroid helping the metabolism. Combining the two technologies allows deeper penetration to the subcutaneous fat layer, and the combined heat generated keeps the treatment area stimulated for up to 24 hours. The typical applicator for this treatment hovers over the body, and the

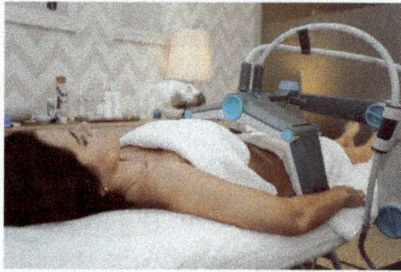

technician will cover any area of the body that is not or cannot be treated. Once the machine is turned on, the technician can leave the room while checking on the client periodically, then returning when the treatment time is complete. The treatment areas focus more on the trunk of the body, buttocks, and thighs.

The number of treatments averages six for the ideal client. Clients with more fat to lose will require more sessions. When you google the average cost of treatment with a machine similar to the UltraSlim is $500 per session for the entire stomach area and possibly the upper thigh area. This depends on the height of your client.

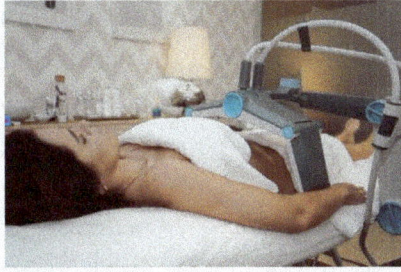

If using an off-brand the price may vary and be a little less. If you select a machine with multiple technologies, or as we call them modalities on one machine that includes infrared light and red light therapy, you would average $180 to $250 a session per treatment area, the treatment area with this type of machine is based on time.

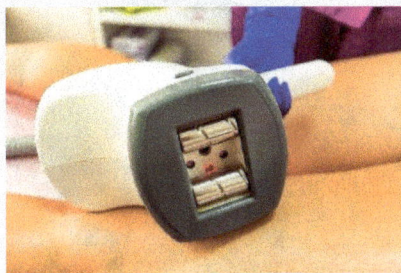

The manufacturer and trainer will provide you with the minimum and maximum treatment times per area. For example, this could be 40 to 60 minutes with the stomach and flanks, and this machine requires the technician for hands-on treatment.

We will cover electromagnetic muscle stimulation; and ultrasound cavitation is the final technology to review. **Electromagnetic Muscle Stimulation** is designed to build muscle through electromagnetic pulsation. Building muscle this way does break down some unwanted fat (volume). The applicator for this technology typically has large paddles placed flat on the treatment area and buckled around the body to stay in place.

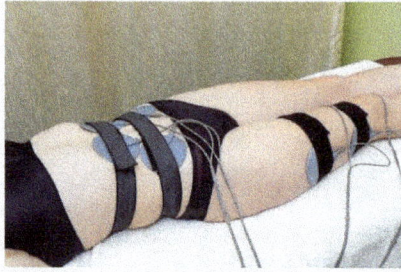

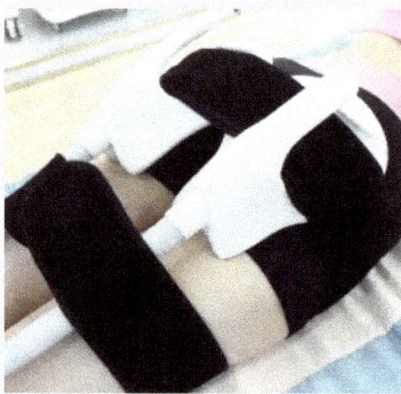

Treatment areas include; the abdomen, buttocks, arms, calves, and thighs. Treatments can be provided twice a week; the average is four treatments over two weeks. This treatment is ideal for clients with a low amount of fat to lose. Again, this is ideal for building muscle, with studies showing the muscle built in four sessions can last six months to a year.

The cost per treatment ranges from $400 to $1000 per area and per session. Market research for your area is encouraged to determine price per session and package pricing options.

Our final technology to cover is ultrasound cavitation. **Ultrasound Cavitation** can be performed surgically and non-surgically. Again for this book, we are only discussing non-surgical options. This includes the original broad ultrasound and the newer intensified focused ultrasound (also known as HIFU or Ultherapy.)

BROAD ULTRASOUND HIFU OR ULTHERAPY

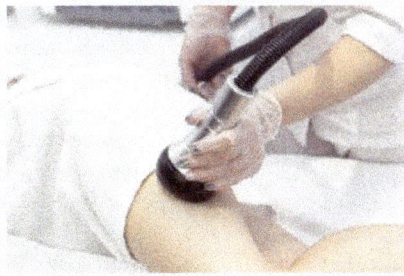

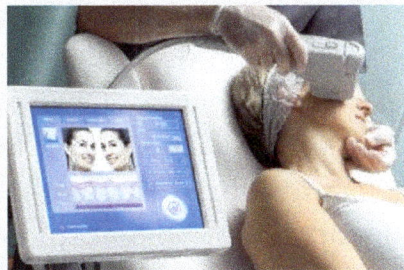

In general, we talk very little about Ultrasound technology. This technology has been around clinically since 1956. Most know ultrasound for how it helps to see inside the body; showing us cysts, tumors, and the joy of new life, babies.

With adjusting the frequency of ultrasound to a range of 25 to 40 hertz the waves will not bypass the muscle layer but will be a frequency that toxins attached to the fat cell in the subcutaneous layer can no longer maintain their structure. As a result, it melts subcutaneous fat, bypassing the skin and tissue. Since it does not go past the muscle layer these waves ripple and continue until they dissipate, resulting in melting fat in the treatment area and affecting the surrounding area to a small degree.

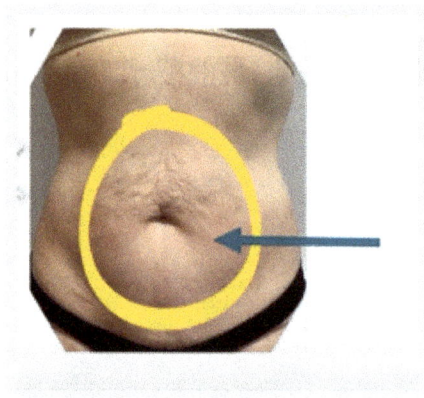

When using broad ultrasound, it is administered through a flat wand-shaped handle onto the body. This type of applicator cannot be left in one spot or affixed to the body. It is required to be placed on the body and kept in constant motion. (Even though the ultrasound bypasses the skin, and tissue, leaving this applicator in one place on the body generates too much energy in one spot, causing excess heat that could blister the skin.) Due to the need for constant movement in the treatment area, clients experience what feels like a hot stone massage. This applicator can come in two sizes. With a small handle for the face, shorter treatment times are needed. A larger handle can be used on other areas of the body. Treatment times with this handle, like on the entire stomach, and can be 40 to 60 minutes of hands-on work by the technician.

Intensified Ultrasound is the same technology; however, the handle uses cartridges.

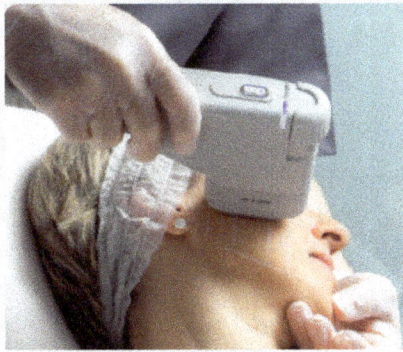

Inside this cartridge the mechanical device emitting the ultrasound wave is submerged in water. A controlled amount of energy is forced through pin size holes that are organized in rows and columns. Some would say it appears similar to the design of the number 12 domino without the line in the middle.

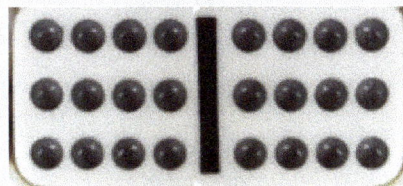

Each row of dots can be spaced closer or farther apart. Your manufacturer and trainer will provide specific instructions on settings.

Broad Ultrasound and Intensified Ultrasound technology can be used on the cheeks, under the chin, arms, bra line, stomach, flanks, buttocks, and thighs. Regarding how many treatments, we will discuss the two separately: Broad Ultrasound studies show for a perfect candidate, six sessions are recommended for optimal results, and they will see additional results for up to three weeks after treatment (provided the client does their self-care.) Treatments can be administered every 3 days (to better explain, on the fourth day after a treatment) or once a week until desired results. Depending on the client's needs, it could be more or less. If the client has more than a couple of inches to lose, they will need more treatments.

Intensified Ultrasound can be used to provide a facelift and body contouring. For a facelift, a client may have 1 to 3 sessions depending on the machine settings, volume in the cheeks/neck area and level of lift needed.

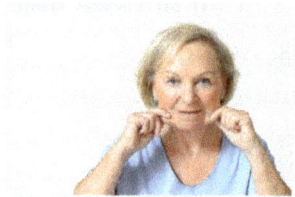

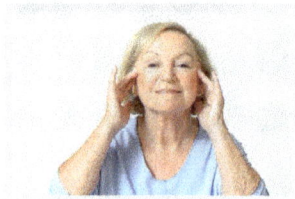

Body contouring with intensified ultrasound can be one session for an ideal client wanting to lose 1 to 2 inches.

Please note the treatment area with this technology is typically 2"x8", so targeting the source of the problem is essential to achieve these results in 1 to 2 sessions, and

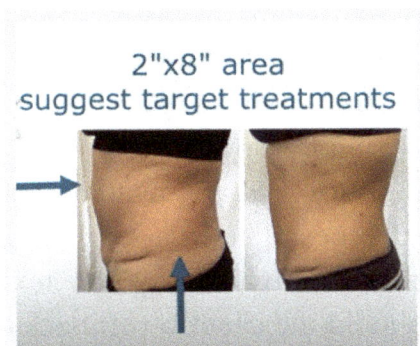

for example can very well be four areas just for the stomach. Clients wanting more than a couple of inches will have an increase in sessions and treatment areas. Your manufacturer and trainer will provide these treatment areas in more detail. The cost of this treatment varies depending on the market threshold, providers in the area, and what equipment grade it is "registered as" with the FDA. Broad Ultrasound services are typically provided in treatment times varying at a minimum of 40 minutes for $125 up to $200 and 60 minutes for $175 to $300.

Intensified Ultrasound services, depending on if it's Hifu or Ultherapy, can range approximately from $250 an area to $500 area. The approximate treatment area size is slightly over 2" x 8". This completes the overview of the six types of technologies in the non-surgical contouring industry; Cryolipolysis, Laser Lipolysis, Radio Frequency, Combined Infrared & Red Light therapy, Electromagnetic, and Ultrasound. Be sure to do your own research on the benefits of reducing body fat and increasing muscle mass. Hopefully, this has provided you with the details to help you with your particular practice and what technologies you may want to use in your spa.

As promised, we will review how to help explain The Difference between surgical and non-surgical. This may sound simple; however, as you continue in this industry, you will notice several providers and technicians do not know the difference. The non-surgical options we have reviewed in this book break away the toxins leaving the healthy fat cell; should the client revert back to an unhealthy lifestyle, they will gain weight proportionally. Non-surgical treatments last as long as the client maintains a balanced, healthy lifestyle, managing stress is also helpful.

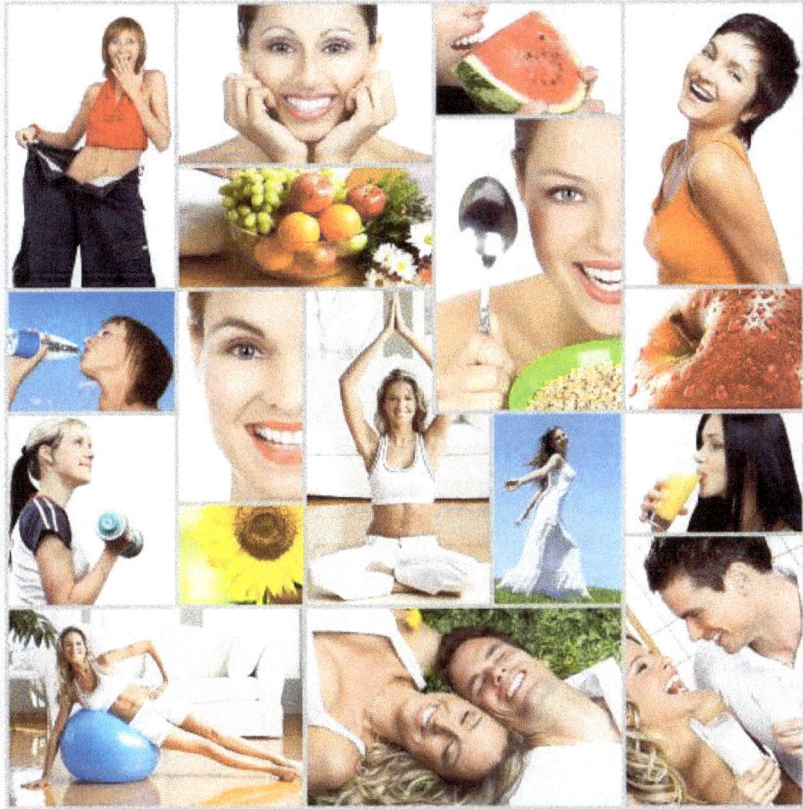

If not, as with surgical and non-surgical, you can begin to gain weight the day after either procedure. Surgical Liposuction will physically suck out the toxins and the healthy fat cells. This process does not leave the healthy fat cells behind. That's why you don't see subcutaneous fat return to the area that received the invasive liposuction.

Toxins such as carbs, sugar, and alcohol, are bound together by stress and cortisol. The developing fat will find other places to attach themselves in the body. That's why those who have surgical liposuction may experience increased fat in other places such as hips, arms, or back. In their minds, these areas become the new problem areas instead of under-standing the need for a balanced diet and active lifestyle. Additionally, if you are let's say 20 or 30 lbs. overweight, most plastic surgeons will request you lose 5 to 10 lbs. before they will perform surgical liposuction. They know there is visceral fat they cannot remove. The patient has to do the work. The weight loss also gives the plastic surgeon more confidence in their health during surgery and the successful long-term look of their work.

I've provided a simple CHART COMPARING SURGICAL VS NON-SURGICAL CONTOURING:

Ultrasound & Radio Frequency	Coolsculpting (Cryo-Freezing)	Sculpsure (Laser Lipo)	Emsculpt (High Frequency)	Sonabello / Injection Lipolysis / Liposuction	Surgical Liposuction and/or Skin Removal
Non Invasive	Non Invasive	Non Invasive	Non Invasive	Invasive treatments	Invasive treatments
30-60 min sessions	43 - 60 min session	30 - 60 min session	30 - 60 min session	Times Vary	Times Vary- 1 - 4 hours
$140 - $400 a session	$300 per handle	$300 per handle	$750 an area	$2500 Sonabello per area $300 injection Lipo an area $3200 Liposuction (per area)	$3,000-20,000 Varies: Volume of fat & skin removal
Multiple sessions until desired results	Multiple sessions until desired results	Multiple sessions until desired results	Multiple sessions until desired results		Visits: How many areas for approved surgery. Minimum: 3 visits (consultation, surgery, follow up)
Treatment areas: Face, Neck, Biceps, Bra Line, Back, Stomach, Flanks, Buttocks, Legs	Treatment areas: Chin - 1 handle Stomach - 4 handles Flanks - 2-4 handles Legs - 2-4 handles	Treatment areas: Stomach- 2-6 handles Flanks - 2-6 handles Legs - 2-12 handles	Treatment areas: Stomach - upper / lower Flanks Back Legs - Inner / Outer Bi-ceps	Number of visits vary Treatment areas: Face, Neck, Arms, Bra Line, Back, Stomach, Buttocks, Thights, Legs	Treatment areas: Face, Neck, Arms, Bra Line, Back, Stomach, Buttocks, Thights, Legs
Treatments: Intense Ultrasound (face/neck only) is once every 60 days	Treatments: 1 area can be treated every 6-8 weeks	Treatments: 1 area can be treated every 4 weeks	Treatments: 1 area twice a week	Healing: Sonabello - Anesthesia, healing entry sites, possible scaring	Healing: Surgical incision, visible scarring, regaining mobility, ensure lymphatic system works properly throughout the body
Broad Ultrasound (melt fat) 1x a week				Injection Lipolysis- Multiple injections in one area, possible scaring, 1-4 visits	
Radio frequency, Infrared, Vacuum massage (melting/ tightening) 1x a week	Non Invasive Treatments: (Ultrasound, Radio Frequency, CoolSculpting, Sculpsure, Emsculpt, etc.) No downtime, No time off work required, No additional costs , No prescribed medications, No scarring			Liposuction - Anesthesia, scaring, healing	Extra costs: Prescribed medications, medical bandages, time off work 1 - 6 weeks

4

CLIENT CONSULT AND COMMUNICATION; OBTAIN AND RETAIN YOUR CLIENTS

ANOTHER KEY to successfully treating your clients is to know how to communicate with them and provide results. The Client questionnaire is vital in assessing what you can do for each client and ensuring their safety. On each client questionnaire, you should list any contradictions in the treatments you provide and understand how they affect the body; chapter 1 of this book gives you a good overview. However, your manufacturer and trainer should provide the list of contractions for the machine they sold to you.

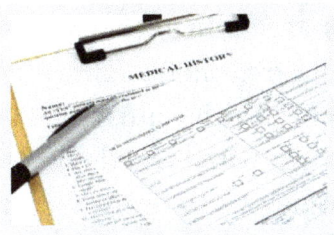

Upon review of the client's questionnaire answers, make sure you confidently explain that the honesty of their answers ensures they maintain their current level of health throughout the treatments and get the maximum results.

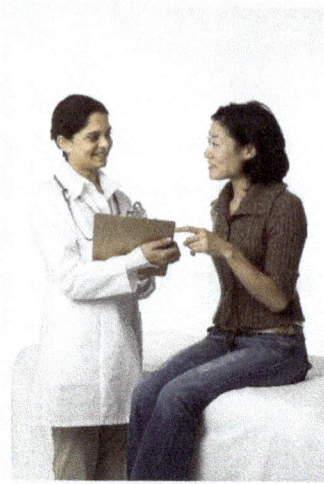

As you review the questionnaire with the client, listening is a solid skill set to have and key. Be sure to listen if the client has something to say during the consultation. It could be of value and could gain information that was accidentally omitted from the intake form. A critical phrase you might hear them say is, "this might be a stupid question." Please reassure them there are no stupid questions regarding treatment on their body, and could lead to health concerns they forgot to include.

A red flag I have encountered is when a client gets defensive. When a client discusses their current health and wants you to tell them what the healthy levels should be for example, triglycerides or cholesterol, to compare their recent results. I take the side of caution and ask when they went in for their last tests. If within a year, I ask, have they been consistent on their medications for six months with no changes? If the client continues to be defensive or unclear, I ask them to please get in touch with their doctor to confirm the results and get written permission to have the treatment. Knowing that being confident is a client's current health status is valuable. Also, you will want to comfort them with your desire to ensure they stay healthy during treatment; you want to get optimal results without potential health risks.

Additionally, safeguarding that you have accurate information reduces the risk of a health complaint, lawsuit, or worse. Remember, any time you doubt a client's honesty, continued defensiveness, or are unclear, have them get a doctor's approval before treatment. The quality client you are looking for will appreciate you putting them first. A client who gets upset is a potential risk you want to avoid taking.

Another component of client communication we will review is determining how to treat areas to achieve the client's wants. Typically the manufacturer and trainer will show you how to divide the treatment areas; however, I want to add another element that is not reviewed by most; how what's above affects below on the body, the joy of gravity. Yes, it applies to non-surgical contouring.

Let's review some examples; When a client walks in and asks to reduce or lift the lower stomach (sometimes the following Urban words like; the apron, or dunlap,) looking at what is above the requested treatment area can affect the success of your results. If they have fat (volume) above the lower stomach, I will ask permission to show them how treating the area above will benefit and maximize their results

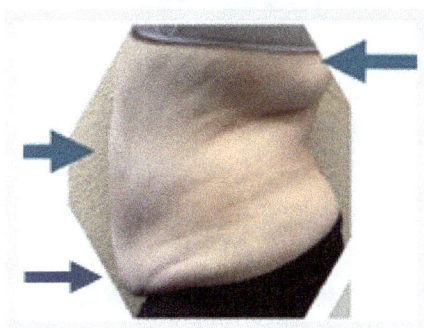

(QUICK note, please get permission to touch the client, DO NOT just grab their body, as this is a very private and personal choice to allow you to see their most vulnerable self-conscious area of their body). Once permission is granted, I politely grab hold of the upper stomach and lift, showing them how it affects the lower stomach area in the mirror. From a provider's standpoint, yes this means you can treat more areas and that increases your sales. For the client, they will get closer to their goal and the knowledge that only treating the requested area will not achieve optimal results. The "above affects below" approach is one of the many ways to review the body in what is affecting the treatment area.

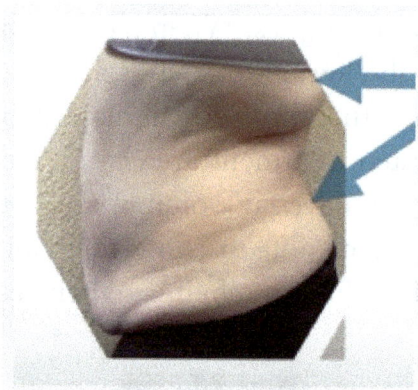

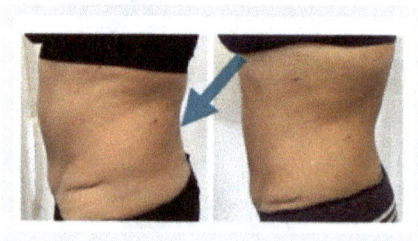

It is understood that we gain volume on the back side, and with the design of our body, it only expands so far back there before it starts pushing the fat forward. So when reviewing treatment requested for the front of the body, it can benefit results to see if they have any fat (or volume) on the backside. Again get permission to touch a clients' body if you are working your way around their bodies and lift to see if other areas affect the treatment area.

In assessing treatments for the face, if the client wants to eliminate or improve the jowls, you will want to evaluate the face from the upper cheeks down to determine if they have a structural loss from reduced collagen and elastin production.

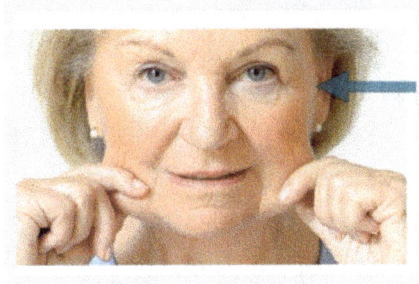

Now you could just treat the jowls but if the support from above is lacking, you would need to treat above, to help fully lift the jowls strengthening the overall structure. A great practice exercise for you before consulting patients would be to start by examining your body in the mirror. Let's look at your lower back and the top of the buttocks area. Place your hands on the lower back or flanks, then lift.

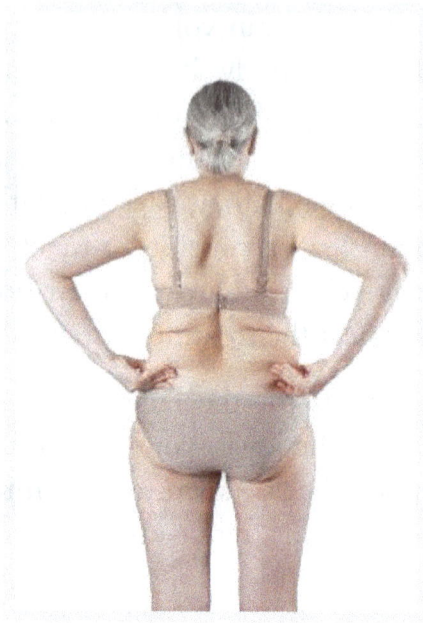

You may notice that the lower back and butt will have a more lifted appearance if you have some tightening or volume to lose. This may also affect the top part of the upper thigh, depending on how much loose skin is there. If you try this example on the stomach, the same concept applies if you lift the top of the stomach the lower stomach and top of the upper thigh are affected. Sometimes you can see an additional difference in the upper thigh when you lift only the lower stomach. These are just some great examples of how what above affects below, how what is in the back affects the front, and tips on how to show clients the best way you can optimize results for the requested treatment area.

When determining how many sessions a client may need, I first want to explain the typical marketing you see for non-surgical body contouring. Most of this marketing is based on their ideal client. This ideal client is someone who is looking to lose a few inches and would generally receive the average recommended number of treatments. Even though some manufacturers don't explain how many sessions are necessary for clients who are looking to lose more than 2 inches, the directions they typically give is to have the client come in for the recommended minimum. Then strategically expecting when the client sees results, they will just keep coming in. Using that strategy, even the best clients who understand the process will start to get discouraged. Clients need a goal or a level of realistic expectations. This is why when I review with a client who wants more than 1 to 2 inches gone I explain to them, "a little more or a little less treatment may be needed," and "everyone responds differently, but we are both striving for the same goal, and that is getting results." Due to my own personal story is why I make the extra effort to provide this information and support, I know how this process feels.

No professional should give up on the client during their first consultation or discourage them when they want to healthily look their best. Later in this book, I will discuss a better approach for these clients.

We will now review the value of discussing with a client, the difference between fine-tuning, budging stubborn areas, and helping with weight loss to determine how many sessions. Fine-tuning is where a client is in excellent shape, maybe returned from a trip, and had overindulged. This type of client may be a one or two-session client. Budging stubborn areas, this client is generally healthy but may have additional factors affecting them; this could include not being aware of the proper exercise, age, or hormone changes. This client will most likely be at least the minimum treatments based on the recommendations by the manufacturer. With the minimum sessions required by the manufacturer, clients on a weight loss journey, and clients with several inches to lose in one area, I inform the client they will see changes, which will help you get through your first 30 days.

From my professional experience, I recommend ultrasound cavitation for this process, as the treatment can be given once every three days or once a week. This technology provides the weekly encouragement a client needs and carries them through the first six weeks of their journey. Often, a client will ask about more treatments beyond the recommended. This is an excellent opportunity to keep the ball rolling, and they can go up to 10 weeks at a once-a-week treatment. After that, they continue on their own, and depending on how much weight they want to lose, they can come in every 5 lbs of weight loss to help budge through plateaus, and if you provide skin tightening, you can minimize excess loose or sagging skin. As described previously in chapter one, as we age, the skin is less responsive without receiving some external support. Below is a photo of an actual client who lost 80lbs and then came into my spa. This client agreed to coming in once a week for six months. With having two children, she could not have downtime from surgical options. We set up a schedule for alternating ultrasound cavitation, melting, and skin tightening to assist her in reaching her goals.

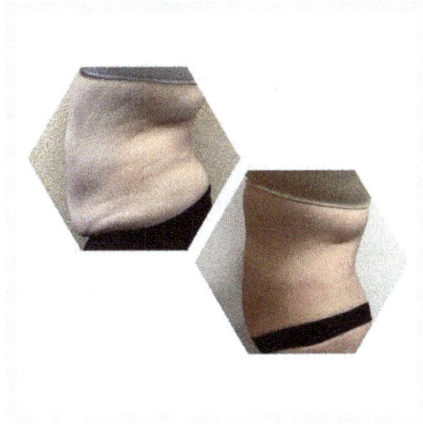

You might be asking why I didn't recommend the cryolipolysis or laser lipo options for the rest of her weight loss journey. With my research and experience, cryolipolysis is once every six weeks, and the laser is once every four weeks. Most clients on a weight loss journey have higher success when touching base at a weekly appointment (a form of self-accountability). Clients can still be successful with other non-surgical options. And it is always possible that you or someone else will create a plan that could work, keeping a client encouraged and understanding the process. As we have reviewed, all treatments work with educated providers. Understanding everything that affects the client's body is a key component to properly treating and achieving optimal results. One-and-done may be a surgical option, and surgery does not always give the final look that clients have in their minds. Everything else, non-surgical, is a series of treatments until desired results are achieved and then maintenance mode. Maintenance mode, be it with their balanced diet and activity and maybe once or twice a year non-surgical touch-ups depending on their lifestyle choices.

Provider and client consistency is another key – Yes, another great analogy; Consistency is like the oil change for your vehicle. If you do not change the oil regularly and have routine checkups, they will not get the optimal performance of their automobile. Staying consistent with treatment until desired results optimizes them and the longevity of retaining those results. Determine the need and or longevity of support. Reviewing a client's overall health and habits of a client will help assess the starting number of treatments for the client, and the kind of conversational support that might benefit them at each visit. Having conversations with clients at each visit, some may see this as a personal touch they do not want to bother with; I see this as an opportunity to stand out and gain client retention and word-of-mouth referrals by adding this personal element. The type of conversation based on the level of support a client needs is beneficial. This can affect many aspects, including; clients' self-care at home, increased confidence in the providers' skills, and a stronger desire to maintain results and share the details with others.

The type of conversation I recommend is more of a peer listening approach. You would not be giving them guidance. The conversation would allow your client to hear them-selves, acknowledge the good they've done and the tough areas they want to change. Some examples include; for a client starting a weight loss journey during each visit, you could say: How was your week? How do you feel about your food, water, and activity levels? Good - ask for details. Bad – you could ask what they didn't like, how would they like to change it. Finish with, it's a good thing that day is gone, and today we get to focus on moving forward and making better choices. You are doing a fantastic job!

For clients coming in to treat stubborn areas, the same two questions about what is good and what is bad, apply from above. You may also add through this process, they will see results in the first visit and more as they move forward into week four; as this is when the most results will show (no matter which technology they use for treatment.) The reason for adding in this detail is because clients, who are overall healthy, believe the area is small, and think they only need one treatment. After the first session they then wonder why it is not gone and will think the treatment is not working. With stubborn areas they may need two to four treatments. The stubborn area is usually due to not choosing the proper exercise for the target area, age, or hormones. A reminder from the previous chapter, after the age of 35 or having children, our hormones start changing and our body is less responsive.

Clients that are coming in for skin tightening. Again the same first two questions apply, and you could add that going through this process, they may see minor results in the first visit and more as they progress. For example, suppose a client has had loose skin for over 10 years, in addition to general aging, hormones, and lifestyle factors. In that situation, we would need to remind the skin cells to do their job.

A relatable example for skin tightening would be for example, similar to when you leave the light on in your car, and it drains the car battery. The battery is still good; it just needs a jump start. Sometimes the jumpstart process takes a minute or so to recharge, depending on the age of the battery. But once fully charged, it's good to go, same with the skin. As with car batteries, they eventually need to be replaced. We cannot replace our skin, however, we do occasionally need touch up treatments.

Another way to help keep a client encouraged and sometimes yourself as a provider, we are going to review photos and why they matter, the before and after. First and foremost, ensure that your consent form for treatment includes consent for taking photos. Also, it is strongly suggested to add a disclaimer about photos being used for marketing purposes. To help with client consent, you can add to the disclaimer that as long as the photos have no distinguishing marks on the client, such as tattoos. If a client still gives permission, have them write their authorization on the form, and you both initial. For photos, choose a quality camera with a high pixel count; this will provide clear quality photos to show clients and use for marketing. I decided to purchase the Apple iPad because it had the number one quality camera on the market, on-screen grid feature and excellent storage space. Technology changes and improves every year, be sure to do your research or someone to help. If you are like me and need to communicate between different apps and technology, like apple to android, I found an app that will help. It is called "photo-transfer". It works nicely to transfer photos when both devices are on the same Wi-Fi.

When taking photos, you need to have a designated, clean area to take explicit images, this saves you time and adds consistency. The designated area should have a clean background, even if you have to hang a non-patterned curtain on the wall and there's no window behind it. I recommend you use the grid feature for all images (if available on your device). Also, mark on the floor where you want your client to stand, where you stand and where you do not want the lens of the camera to go past. This will help keep a consistent photo depth and size, saving time when collaging client treatments. You want your photos to be as close to the same depth/distance and size so it is more evident to clients when they see them.

Positioning clients in photos: Always take a front photo and a photo from both sides. When you create the collage photos, you will see in the client results that they may change vertically in one visit and then horizontally on the next visit. This means that the skin is lifting vertically, and horizontally is melting. The alternating between visits is the body catching up.

For some clients, measuring after every visit is helpful. Just be sure to measure the same spot each time; typically this is through the middle of the treatment area.

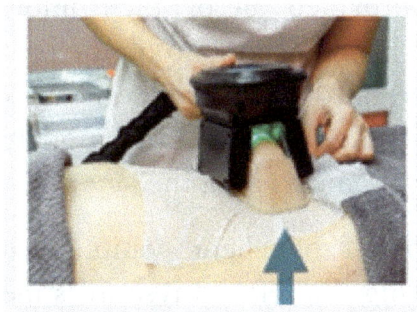

(Measuring example: with a coolsculpting treatment, you would place a handle on the upper and lower stomach, shown in the picture. With using two handles; that is two measurements. The measuring tape would go around the body and place in the middle of where the handle was put on the body for treatment. The manufacturer and trainer should provide the before and after measuring guidelines.)

When presenting progressive treatment photos: I inform clients that during their first visit, there will be two photos, a before and a right after photo taken and shown in a collage picture. Then going forward, we will only take an after picture. For each visit following, you will use the after photo from the previous treatment and the after photo from that day for the current collage. When their series of treatments are complete, I make the collage of their before treatments with the after treatment photo of their last visit. With that said, sometimes, if a client's treatment plan goes past four weeks, a client who sees themselves everyday can get discouraged and stuck in their head that maybe this is not working. At that point, I will create a collage photo of the before treatments with the after photo of week four. This does boost their confidence and commitment to the process. (Note; sometimes this collage may tell you that the client has not provided all of their information. If the provider has not been keeping up on the per session conversations, it will be hard to determine if the client has been using the treatments as a crutch to their goals, and not doing the aftercare requirements at home.)

Another component of client communication and their success is reviewing the referral resources mentioned earlier in this book. The additional assistance your clients may need to ensure long-term success may be something mentioned in this chapter. This list of resources includes a nutritionist, naturopathic doctor, personal trainers, spiritual reiki, and lymphatic massage therapists. (Note; you may find more resources as more research becomes available.) Now let's briefly review why these resources add value;

Nutritionists can provide insight into how food is connected to emotions and stress. They can also provide knowledge on how to balance their diet for continued success.

A naturopathic doctor can test hormones, cortisol levels, and digestive issues that all may be part of what is preventing their weight loss, and other possible underlying health concerns. How this is relatable to non-surgical contouring is my personal story. At age 41, I discovered that my IUD had eliminated my hormones, causing my cortisol levels to skyrocket. Also, add the stress of moving to a different state and starting my business in Colorado. I gained over 9 lbs. in less than three months and could not understand why! After talking with a friend, I went to a naturopath to test my hormones. The results, my hormones were bottomed out, constantly spiking cortisol, and digestive issues from the candida buildup in my system (it is possible the antibiotics from my surgeries contributed to this buildup). Just as I started to fix these issues, I became severely sick in February. Then a surprise in March, we had the Covid quarantine and a worldwide shutdown. My stress was through the roof, but with the help of my naturopath doctor my hormones are getting back on track, my digestive system is better and my weight loss journey is progressing.

Personal trainers allow learning exercises most beneficial for a client's journey. This might seem like a logical option to consider for you might be a foreign thought to your client. Understanding exercise basics and gaining a routine, which best suits their life, by going to a certified and experienced trainer for even a short time can give them a lifetime of health benefits.

Spiritual Reiki is an alternative spiritual option. The world is divided on the subject; some nonbelievers, borderline believers and others that are entirely into the practice. For the nonbelievers and borderline believers, I approach the subject delicately and give them my favorite example from one of my clients. An example; this method in reference to stomach contouring; focuses on the shape of the belly and lack of results. In Spiritual Reiki the lack of results can be from blocked energy.

A prior client of mine wanted to reduce the volume in her stomach. During the consultation the stomach was round and firm to the touch. I asked my client how her work and home environment were; for her, work was her primary source of stress. I asked whether you have negative coworkers in the office. Immediately she responded oh my word, yes. Does the air feel heavy when she's in the room? "Yes," she replied. Do you ruminate over it when you get home? "Yes, sometimes, and I can't sleep. I dread going in the next day," she said. So, I asked if she had ever considered energy work by a trusted reiki provider. In short, she had heard about it but wasn't sure if it really worked. I explained that I was not an expert; however, my basic understanding of the chakras and energy involved with the stomach is where we can hold emotions and stress. Clearing those chakras and learning to block a negative person's energy may provide significant benefits during treatment and your overall daily health. The client came in the following week; I noticed her stomach was softer. I asked what she was doing differently since her last visit; she had gone into a Spiritual Reiki provider. For the first time in 2 sessions her stomach had not only softened she continued to see results during each visit. From examples like this during my career, I believe in energy work and its benefits. You may not, but your clients might, and you must remember that this process is about their journey.

Moving on with Lymphatic massage therapists, as we discussed earlier, the lymphatic flowing properly is one of the critical components to flushing out the toxins of the body as well as helping with Cellulite and is very helpful after a client has had surgery anywhere near their lymphatic system (such as a tummy tuck or breast alteration) the lymph system can be compromised. This technique has proven to help many regain a positive effect on their health, weight loss, reduced stress, and ultimately maximizing their results. The research is fascinating and I encourage you to read more on lymphatic massage benefits.

This wraps up discussing the value of alternative resources that you could recommend. Remember, if you do not believe in these alternatives, your client might, and they are the ones who may need this information to achieve their best self. Additionally, showing this added personal touch and making these professional connections increase your word-of-mouth referrals from both the professional and the client.

Some additional bonus material that may help your clients and marketing strategy, we are going to review the well-known mommy pouch, belly types and liposuction aftercare.

The well-known Mommy Pouch: Traditional curriculums do not provide the complete knowledge on how to help mothers after childbirth, take care of their skin.

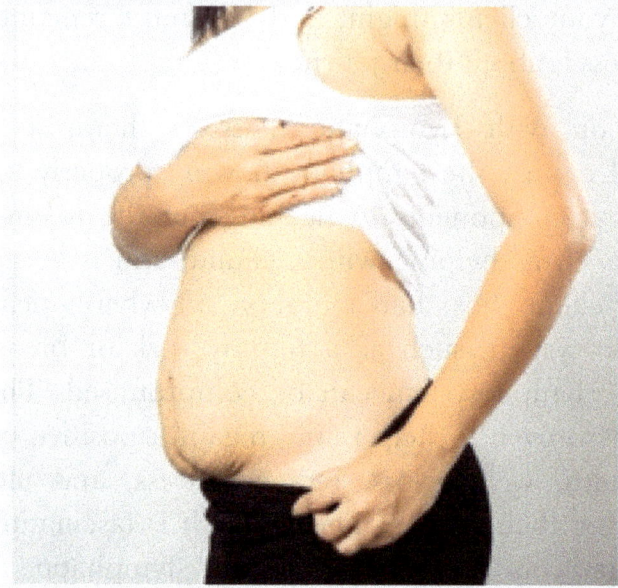

Most recommendations to resolve the unwanted pouch are "mommy makeovers" tummy tucks. However, with my clients, I found that if they wear a semi-firm compression tank after birth (adjustments may need to be made for the breast area of the top, or purchase a top that only goes over the stomach), a light exfoliation of the body, and apply approved topical hydrating oil after showering, in an upward motion. This at home recommendation assists with stimulating the skin to tighten during the afterbirth healing process. Then after they have stopped breast feeding, they have the option to combine the homecare with non-surgical options such as radio frequency and ultrasound technology. The combination would diminish, if not eliminate the need for a surgical solution. (My favorite compression tanks are from Maidenform.

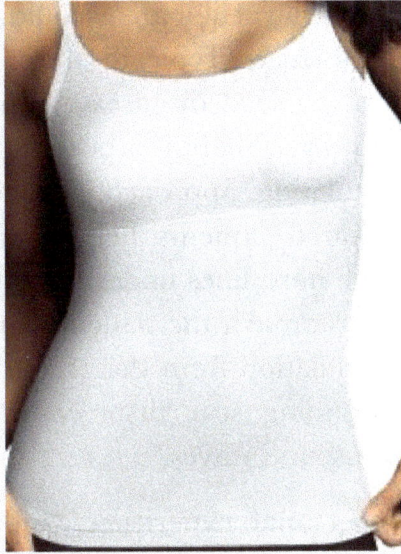

You can measure the client by focusing on the waist measurement only, review the sizing chart, and select a size smaller for the client. Most importantly, instruct the client to step in and step out of the top, never go over the shoulders. This is because the material typically doesn't stretch far enough without causing shoulder strain.)

You may wonder why I said the client would start non-surgical treatments after breastfeeding. This relates to our review of the breakdown of fat cells: how they affect the lymphatic system, cholesterol and blood pressure. Because of this process it would also affect the breast milk as it is another way toxins exit the body and you would not want to feed those toxins to your new baby.

Another tip in regards to helping clients who have surgical liposuction; what you may not know about traditional liposuction, if the surgeon is not using ultrasound technology during the procedure, hardened areas could form where the liposuction was performed. Typically they will recommend to their patients to massage the area during healing. This can be effective; however, there is a possibility the area may need a more stimulating approach. Research has found ultrasound cavitation treatments helpful after liposuction. The results show the hard lines under the skin to soften and provide the smooth stomach the patient wanted to achieve. In addition, the stimulation from this technology helps with relaxing the surrounding scar tissue with the dissipating massage of the ultrasound waves.

In my research, personal experience, and seeing clients, surgical liposuction does not stimulate the skin to rebuild the collagen and elastin. Typically a surgeon anticipates the patient's skin to tighten on its own. As we have mentioned, that does not happen for everyone.

Also, many times a patient who has had a tummy tuck, will have what we would call a pucker on their sides. This is where the incision ends and can be created by not having lipo with the tummy tuck or fat removed from the flanks.

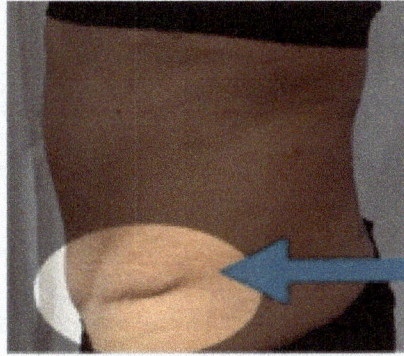

Many surgeons find that having the technology in their office is not a significant financial gain. However, it is a positive gain for nurses and estheticians to increase their income as a separate service for surgical aftercare!

Another tip when assessing a client's needs for optimal results, is recognizing the varying belly shapes and what causes them can help the provider. Studies show there is some insight to caring for clients when you can identify the various shapes of someone's belly. We all understand we cannot please every client or be their one-stop-spa; however, recognizing how we can help or whom to refer them to can help your client select your business for treatment and provide word-of-mouth referrals over the competition. Many online sources will provide additional details and the most up-to-date studies. For this book, we will review the four basics shapes as shown in the image to get a general idea:

The Alcohol belly; typically created by alcohol consumption. The belly shape will have a hard round protruding shape.

The Hormonal belly; typically created by an imbalance of the body's hormones. A larger lower abdomen and increased weight on the lower back

The Stressed Out belly; typically created by the increase in cortisol levels in the body. The upper belly is larger than the lower, almost a B shape.

The Mommy belly; created after giving birth and possible hormone issues. The B shape with the lower abdomen larger and pulling more downward in front.

Having an idea of what is causing the shape may help you decide if referring the client to an outside source may be helpful for you to provide optimal results.

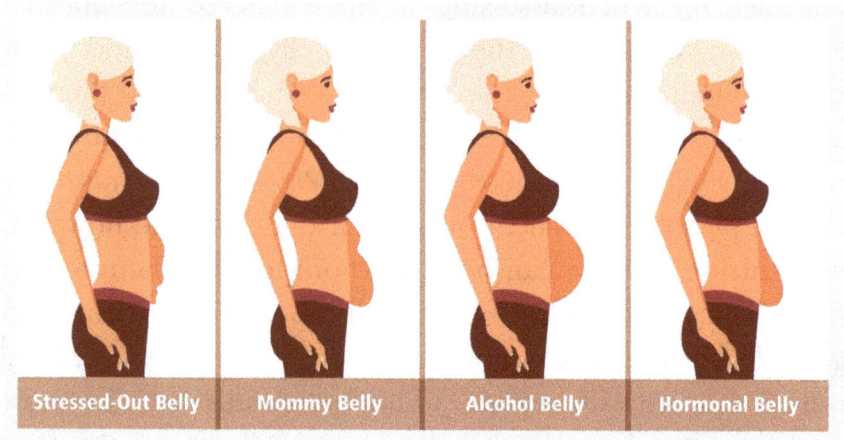

Stressed-Out Belly   Mommy Belly   Alcohol Belly   Hormonal Belly

5

CLIENT CONSULT AND COMMUNICATION; OBTAIN AND RETAIN YOUR CLIENTS

IN TODAY'S WORLD, there is a growing trend with Botox and cosmetic fillers. This chapter will review the basic understanding of Botox, fillers and how they compare to non-surgical treatments.

Botox: (Which affects the contractions of facial muscles) is a drug made from the same toxin that causes life-threatening food poisoning called botulism. Doctors have been known to treat some health issues and temporarily smooth facial wrinkles by weakening or paralyzing the facial muscle with small doses of this toxin. How it works: The injection of Botox blocks specific chemical signals from the nerve endings that communicate with the facial muscles. As the Botox starts to bind with the connection point between the nerve and muscle is why results typically begin within a few days but may take up to two weeks. The injection usually lasts 3 to 6 months, depending on the patient and if they have had prior Botox injections.

Fillers: (Affects the Dermis layer of the skin), A gel-type substance is injected into the dermal layer of the skin, hence the name Dermal filler. How it works: The filler is injected into the dermis layer to increase volume and provide an instantly fuller appearance on the face, diminishing or eliminating lines on the face. Although the injected filler takes approximately four weeks to integrate (settle) into the tissue fully, it can last six to twelve months (some products may last longer). Therefore, manufacturers typically recommend checking fillers at least every twelve months.

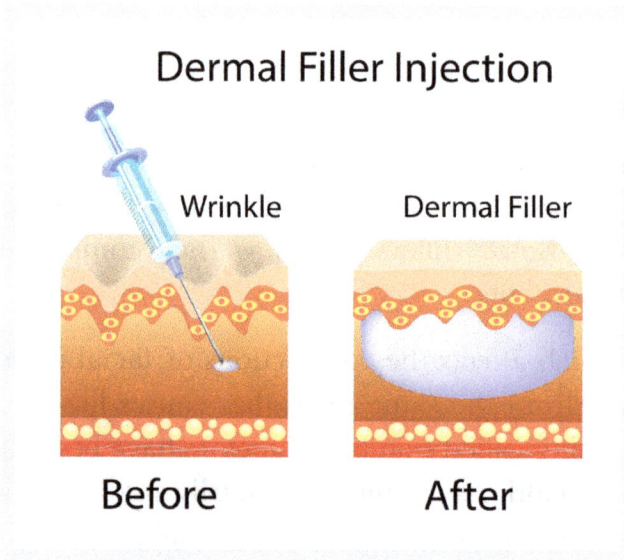

Dermal Filler Injection

Wrinkle   Dermal Filler

Before   **After**

Non-surgical Contouring: Intensified Ultrasound (affects the Dermis and SMAS layer of the skin) How it works: Releasing a highly concentrated ultrasonic energy into the skin causes a precise thermal coagulation (heat generated disruption) points at the base of the SMAS layer. Delivering tiny deposits of focused ultrasound energy, it precisely heats a specific location in a short period. Your skin responds by stimulating the tissue to produce new compact collagen fibers. These treatments lead to a natural and gradual tightening/improvement of your skin's elasticity and firmness. As the skin tightens, wrinkles become less visible. In addition, the texture of the skin improves, becoming smooth, shiny and firm.

New collagen takes four months to produce; this treatment accelerates, and shows some results immediately and works up to 30-90 days.

Radio Frequency (affects the Dermis layer of the skin) How it works: Distributing a high frequency of alternating current that will heat the dermis layer of the skin. The heat generated stimulates collagen production to improve the appearance of wrinkles and sagging skin. After one treatment, some results are noticeable right away and can take up to four months to take full effect and can last up to six months. Depending on the changes needed or wanted, the client may need a series of treatments before noticing results. After a final treatment they will continue to improve over the next few months, and with proper skin care, could last for 2 to 3 years.

6

BOTOX, FILLERS, AND HOW THEY COMPARE TO NON-SURGICAL TREATMENTS

MARKETING TIPS; here is a broad overview of some suggestions. Most individuals getting into the non-surgical body contouring industry are either adding to an already existing practice, opening a medical spa business, or wanting to be in the industry and work at a medical spa.

Those adding to their practice already have relationships with clients who trust their recommendations and treatments, so marketing to them is straightforward, or so it seems. An example of what might happen is the existing practice may believe the client is thinking they won't have to find another person to trust; the practice is becoming a one stop shop. However, this doesn't guarantee the clients will be 100% on board. With the staff knowing what is available in the industry and how to answer their questions about how your machine and prices compare is treasurable. This shows the client that you want to continue quality services because you took the time to gain additional knowledge, so they don't have to shop around and compare.

We will now go into more detail and add on to the marketing ideas we previously discussed in exciting existing clients and capturing the interest of new clients.

For example, Surgical Aftercare is fine-tuning the areas surgery doesn't reach, (such as the tummy tuck side pucker or the upper belly bulge, and smoothing liposuction tracks) and stimulating the skin for better movement and tightening after liposuction.

Marketing points for clients who want to start a weight loss journey:

- Acknowledge the first 30-day struggle
- They will get motivated and stay that way
- Seeing the external results by the end of 30 days
- You can add a plan for them to come back every 5 lbs to tighten the skin
- Push through plateaus and keep momentum

When starting a weight loss journey; the client has found a self-care plan to start at home and combined with treatments they can see in the first 30 days, they melt the visceral fat around the organs and the non-surgical treatment melts the subcutaneous fat helping to give the shape of the body they are working towards.

You can also consider community outreach options when marketing. Touch base with local salons, personal trainers, health coaches, nutritionists, naturopaths, and travel agents. You can extend to them a discounted introductory service and referral discount only available to them for paying client referrals. I mention these sources because they have a client base they see regularly who are possibly seeking your services. To help you understand how they can be a valuable contact here are some of the conversations that occur;

"If only my face would look as good as my hair."

"I'm struggling to stay motivated; I'm just not seeing the change fast enough."

Personal trainers, health coaches, nutritionists, naturopaths who might refer clients to you know diet and exercise doesn't always get rid of stubborn areas or help loose skin. If they are not aware, you can share the reasons why our skin doesn't always retract on its own after weight loss and seeking this non-surgical option will give them results, boost confidence and keep the mutual client on track. Being in the self-care business we are focused on helping our clients reach their goals in safe, positive and encouraging ways.

Travel agents may be a good resource because in conversations the client may joke that with an all-inclusive trip they just might overindulge. Knowing about your services might help the travel agent close the deal by referring your services for when they return.

All the tips we've just discussed apply to those just starting out and who still need a client base.

When you do not have a client base where you're located does affect how you market. Some providers may experience the differences between bigger cities vs. smaller towns. In bigger cities, you definitely want to get your ad visible and seen often. Showing your business is clean, professional, caring and focused on providing the max results for each client. In these areas, social media ads are quite effective and the community outreach we mentioned can be even more important when you are starting out with no client base. If you are in a bigger city and have a larger budget, for example, you can maximize your exposure through television ads and billboards.

Learning about what is important to your community, no matter what size the city, has value. This one significant factor put me in a winning position. How the community prefers to interact and support each other allows your business the grand opportunity to gain their trust and boost your business awareness community-wide. This is where word-of-mouth referrals can start to explode.

Starting a business in a small to medium size town without a client base can be difficult. You will want to create a social media platform on Facebook, Instagram and Twitter, as well as a website. Please ensure that your location is visible and that how to reach you is easily accessible on all sites! Also, connecting with other business professionals as mentioned above will be valuable.

Having started in a medium-sized manufacturing town with little to no marketing budget, I can give my own experience. Everyone in town, even the county, had seen every gimmick, pyramid scheme and the feeling resonated that any service provider in this industry was just out for their money. Besides the marketing education I received in college, I read and watched every educational piece that would tell me how to market to such a rural and ridged town. I even attended a conference that featured one of the top marketing companies in the United States. One of the founders told me I would be better off moving my business to a bigger town and improving my luck based on the unsuccessful social media posts and other information I provided. That where I lived was called a black hole in the marketing world. I was crushed; to me there had to be a way, and I found it.

Even though the concept was simple, it did require some work. The community was huge on events in my particular town and including the county. This includes fundraisers, craft shows, women and wellness expos, county small business expos, you name it. This told me that the community preferred one-on-one experiences, seeing, touching, and talking to each other in person to see what they were truly getting. I signed up for the most relatable events where I provided drawings, and with fundraisers offered gift certificates for silent auctions.

My biggest winners were the women and wellness expos. My giveaway box instructed them to like the business on social media, where I will post the winners in 24 hours and watch for my amazing seasonal specials. The second was fundraisers. This approach allowed me to build awareness with other local business owners and community leaders. Since I supported the same things as others in the community, this helped me gain their trust.

This memory brings up the reminder that when it comes to working on someone's body, you have to remember this journey is personal. Gaining trust is essential and allows for you to retain your client and boost word-of-mouth opportunities.

Many consumers find your services by word-of-mouth, google reviews, and result photos. Unfortunately, some clients can be so self-conscious that they will google providers, pick the number one rated, won't ask questions, they'll just request treatment and go out the door. This client could be your potential lousy review.

After I participated in several online groups where consumers received non-surgical treatments, most of the comments were

"They never told me that,"

"How was I supposed to know,"

"Why didn't they tell me?"

"I didn't get results. Waste of money."

These complaints are unnecessary as long as providers know the nonsurgical technology and how to use it properly. But, again, this goes back to the client communication section of this book. Please review it at least twice to help avoid these comments about your services.

7

MARKETING YOUR BUSINESS; WITH/WITHOUT CLIENTS, LIPO AFTERCARE, MOMMY POUCH CARE

LOOKING to start a Medical spa or already have one and want to ensure you have all the facility requirements? This chapter will provide the details based on the more authoritarian states like California and Florida. We will review: licenses, sales tax and insurance, treatment room requirements for injectable/blood exposure vs contouring, software and payment processor options, equipment recommendations, additional services and why, industry staff's expectations, and a summary of consumables.

Medical Spa Facility requirements:

1. Licenses

- Federal EIN (Employer Identification Number)
- State registration
- Local city or town if they require a business license
- Establishment license for the Non-surgical treatment side of the business
- DORA (Department of Regulatory Agency for your state whom manages licensing and regulations) will provide your local spa requirements
- Professional licenses
- The owner/operator for each state is different for medical spas
- Example: California, a physician will need to be the owner/operator
- Example: Michigan, a physician will need to own the equipment and carry the liability and a separate person can own the business with the physician as the medical director
- Example Colorado, the owner is required to have a medical director to operate the equipment
- (Medical Directors are physicians who are licensed and can prescribe medications for at least ten years)
- All states require procedure technicians to have a license and or a certification to touch the body. (Check with your state for your specific requirements)
- Examples: Esthetician, Massage therapist, Laser Certified, Registered nurses, Physician assistants

(ALWAYS CHECK WITH YOUR STATE REQUIREMENTS!)

- Injectable treatments; usually, a registered nurse
- Laser & Cryolipolysis; esthetician and or registered nurse
- Ultrasound Cavitation; esthetician/cosmetologist, laser certified, massage therapist
- Radio frequency; esthetician/cosmetologist, laser certified, massage therapist (some states; registered nurse)

2. A Sales Tax license is only necessary if you sell a client something tangible property/product.

- Tracking and charging: Payment processor setups allow you to record sales tax collections for state and local tax. Be sure to confirm every year if any changes occur.
- NOTE: some states have; state, county, and city sales tax

3. Insurance:

- Coverage for Medical spa services
- General liability, property insurance, professional liability, and or malpractice
- If employees: Add worker's compensation depending on 1099 or W2 staff, you can discuss with your agent.
- Insurance coverage agency (some options) coverage can range from $160-$800 a year
- Hiscox.com covers all the above

- Ascpskincare.com
- Handsontrade.com
- Elitebeautysociety.com
- Insurebodywork.com

4. Treatment room needs for aesthetic services.

- It depends on the number of rooms; dedicate rooms for specific services to save time shuffling equipment and reduce doubling supply costs.
- A Room for Botox/Fillers, Microneedling, Procell MD Microchanneling; any service that punctures the skin risk of blood exposure
- Treatment bed or table that allows the client to lie down or sit up, bed goes up/down. Searching for a hydraulic massage table or even a dental chair is because injection procedures are administered sitting up, microneedling lying down.
- Make sure the base of the bed is not stabilized by a small cylinder foundation – they are very tipsy!
- An example of a good bed approximately $1,200 to $2000 https://www.spaandequipment.com/ BELLAGE_Electric_Facial_Massage_s pa_Bed_table.html?gclid= EAIaIQobChMI1ObY0v2k7wIVkcDACh2fqQc FEAQYBSABEgKCI_D_BwE

The bed covering for microchanneling or microneedling treatments: Rolled sheet paper covering or stretcher sheets

- Sharps (needle) disposal container in every room these treatments will be performed

- Blood pathogen clean-up kit
- Vinyl and latex gloves (size based on your tech and options due to allergies)
- Refrigerator for injectable storage
- Medical roller tray (at least one drawer, store back-up supplies for quick access)
- Wall cabinets for storage, save floor space and provides easy access for technicians
- At least four feet counter space/floor cabinet.
- A relaxing clean spa feel is easily achieved with one accent wall color and a picture or painting on the wall.
- Body Contouring Treatment Room
- The treatment bed, using a hydraulic massage table versus a stationary bed, minimizes back strain on the technician
- Good Bed example: https://www.spaandequipment.com/Stella-electric-medical-spa-treatment-table-facial-chair-bed.html
- You can start with a massage table and later switch out. Obtain a table that has a high weight threshold (ex: 500 lbs. weight limit)
- Upper wall cabinets for storage and leave floor space for equipment
- Medical roller tray for supplies used during treatment
- Sitting Chair
- Coat/clothes hooks
- Quality device for optimal images and photo storage, clients need to see the progressive change

- Photo wall: designate one plain wall for these photos (In the photo below, the dedicated area is the wall next to the door once it's closed.)
- Mirror for consultation (as a courtesy, so clients can review themselves before leaving)
- Tile floors: I recommend an anti-fatigue mat for each side of the treatment bed, it comes in many colors to blend in with the floor
- Décor ideas are the same as above: The photo example below includes one color wall, scenic painting, an LED fireplace, a clean look, and a textured curtain adding comfort.
- Even with medical-grade treatments, clients still expect some relaxation, comfort and to unwind while they are there. And, it will elevate you from stark medical spas giving them that hospital-feel. (Colors matter; for example, blue promotes trust, peace, and loyalty. Orange sunset tones promote comfort and warmth.
- The sample room has one floor machine and two placed on roller carts. Storage is in upper cabinets and one floor corner cabinet:

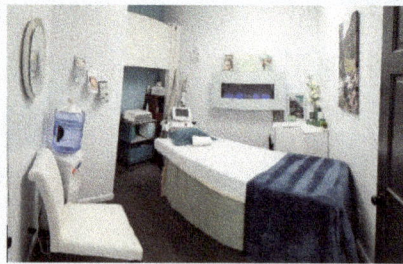

- Facility: Washer and dryer, laundry service (treatment requires a barrier like gel or oil recommendation washable or disposable towels.) I recommend washable towels. It elevates the experience. Especially with gel, paper towels fall apart, removing the gel from treatment areas.

5. Software Recommendations:

- Currently, the software available to the spa industry doesn't capture all needs, however here are some;
- Multi-resource room option
- Package services and tracking
- HIPAA-compliant consent form tracking software
- Accounting reports (have a certified accountant or CPA check the reports it provides to ensure you can report taxes)
- A couple of Spa Software options: Narrowed down to two as they both offer HIPAA compliance, consent forms, scheduling staff and clients, email/text reminders-big for minimizing no-shows and booking specific rooms for specific services. I prefer AestheticsPro; you can schedule a demo to help you decide between software. Note: all pricing mentioned is approximate.
- Meevo 2 $127 − 387 a month (depends on package) https://www.millenniumsi.com/meevo/pricing
- AestheticsPro $109.99 to $229.99 a month (depends on package) https://www.aestheticspro.com/Software-Pricing/
- Vagaro Pro $25 to $85 a month https://sales.vagaro.com/pricing

- Payment processor:
- Meevo, Aesthetics Pro & Vagaro Pro have a point-of-sale system: some have smaller fees per transaction
- The transaction percentage for Visa, MasterCard, Discover, and Amex are sometimes all different and typically have an additional five to ten percent fee.
- Fees or percentages change on amounts processed per month?
- Discount on percentages/fees if credit cards are stored?
- Increase on percentages/fees if the credit card is swiped vs manual card number entered
- Is the payment processor device free? One-time fee?
- These questions will also help you determine how you want to accept payment. Be prepared for clients to pay in cash and have a policy in place for the end of day or the amount in the register to not exceed a certain amount. For example, your treatments might be over $1,000, and they will still pay cash.
- Square is another option that provides a free appointment calendar, free appointment reminder texts, and a website to book appointments.
- Transaction percentage and fees do increase. POS systems have categories they put you in based on your monthly sales transactions. For example, it may be 2.6% +10 cents per swipe/ship/contactless, more for manual entry 3.5% +15 cents, and if they pay online 2.9% +30 cents

- Payment processor device has a free simple swipe. For a POS system, there is a one-time fee.
- Venmo- it's the new trend, and they just created a business account option for clients to pay. The percentage and transaction fees are the lowest I've found at 1.9% +10 cents. It will be an additional account your bookkeeper will need to monitor to reconcile and ensure payment note is added to the transaction to help them update your accounting.
- Customer Financing
- Care credit; Is a credit card for clients. For a MedSpa to qualify typically three different spa services and one product line is needed. They allow your client to use the card with other MedSpas. (Qualifying examples: Waxing, brow/lash tint/perm, facials; each modality used can be a different service.)
- Cherry Financing has been the best and easiest company I've worked with so far. Excellent free marketing tools, periodic email blogs to help grow your business, and fast approval notice via text. Also, when clients apply it doesn't hit their credit report unless they complete a purchase with only your MedSpa. Clients get amazing financing options, posted as a loan on their credit report which helps to build credit versus the hard impact of a credit card. To learn more go to https://refer. withcherry.com/l/0CAVICINC35/

6. Equipment Recommendations:

- There are several machines on the market, and many inexpensive machines do not have clarity on the quality of the machines.
- When purchasing a machine to ensure the client's safety, verify it comes with training and a manual! SAFETY FIRST, then optimizing treatment results, as well as keeping with the integrity of the industry.
- Most manufacturers of contouring equipment in the United States are expensive. They put a lot into marketing the brand name of the machines; below is a suggestion on equipment and approximate pricing comparisons.
- Contouring and other body treatments: Sincoheren is a quality manufacturer located in Beijing, Germany, and has an office in California. Focused on cost-effective machines without sacrificing quality, my extensive research led me to select their machines. I have been pleased with them for the last five years. After two years, I asked to become an independent certified trainer for their machines within the U.S.A. You can contact the company directly for training. They do their best in English however some customers may struggle, so I refer directly to my rep when I recommend the machines I use, aiming for efficiency when it comes to anyone's time. https://www.sincoherengroup.com/products/index_4.html
- I personally know providers in Michigan, Pennsylvania, Florida, Arizona, Colorado, and California that have these machines and love them.

- REP CONTACT: For ordering and good communication, my rep Kelcy Lee is amazing, clear, and very helpful. We trained in person and via zoom. As well as ordered via Whatsapp and the phone for equipment supplies for one of the machines.
- Whatsapp (Secure Communications App for cell phones): +86 187 0134 1926
- Facebook: www.facebook.com/kelcy.lee.39
- Kelcy was promoted at the time of writing this book and may be referring future sales to Brenda Young who is also very good.

7. Additional training in person or for clarification is available separately from certified US trainers like myself. I offer zoom or in-person training on their machines, including client communication, spa business consulting, pricing body treatment areas and sharing techniques I find handy.

- The projected income listed within the equipment recommendation includes anywhere from four to six clients per month with each machine.
- Current in demand services are provided by the following machines; the 808 Diode Laser Hair Removal, Hifu Face and Body Contouring, Ultrasound & RF Face and Body Contouring. Also, the newest trend is the Electromagnetic Muscle Stimulator (such as the EMSculpt machine). Sincoheren would have to provide you with specific pricing; all four machines might run about $

30,000, give or take. With other manufacturers the machines may cost significantly more, see below:

- 808 Diode laser machine, comparable quality, approx. cost $ 39,000
- Hifu Contouring machine, comparable is Ultherapy machine approx. cost $ 80k-100k
- Ultrasound & RF machine, comparable is Velashape approximate cost is $ 17k-26k (VenusLegacy $70k)
- Electromagnetic Muscle Trainer, comparable is Emsculpt, approx. cost $ 250k
- Sincoheren does have several other esthetic machines available, including and not limited to cryotherapy and hydrofacials.
- Why the price difference? You are mainly paying for a brand name, the expense to get the name brand in front of potential clients, and most provide marketing support with the purchase. The big draw for you as a spa owner is that their brand name does draw in clients. However, most clients are just looking for results. You can save money by purchasing an off-brand machine. Compare the machine specifications for quality, and market the results yourself or still spend less with a marketing consultant to get your Med Spa name in the community.
- The estimated cost of the off-brand machines mentioned above ($30,000), does typically include shipping.
- The reason for these specific machines is due to how they work on the body, are effective, and provide great results!

Let's dive into the machines I mentioned to help understand how they can work for you.

A.808 Diode Laser

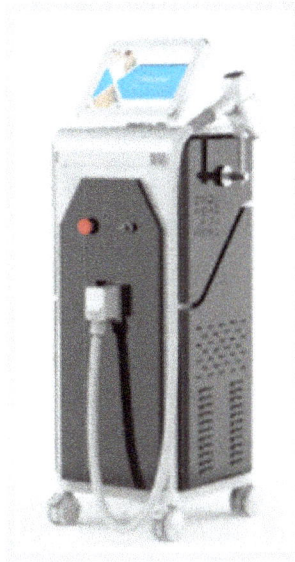

- Benefits of service: Client are in the office every four weeks, with repeat exposure to services and specials
- Target market: Medical professionals and women with PCOS (a hormone issue that causes unwanted hair growth, the treatment doesn't eliminate but minimizes and makes it softer for more comfort and confidence.)
- Pricing and projected income
- Conservative estimation: twelve clients and build from there over twelve months projected gross sales, $60,000 to 102k.

- Pricing for services: $99 to $1000 client packages; startup sale price examples to get clients in the door – bonus, most add more treatment areas.
- X-small area $99-$135 for six treatments
- Small area $169 for six treatments
- Medium area $125-$245 for three treatments
- (regular price medium session is $200, regular multi-session purchase would be 50% off, and intro specials shown are up to 75% off)
- Number of treatments six to ten sessions
- Treatment times:
- X-small: 15min w/client + checkout
- Small: 25min w/client + checkout
- Medium: 40min w/client + checkout
- Large: 50-60min w/client + checkout
- Staffing:
- Technician, depending on your state, minimum an esthetician or registered nurse and an employee under the physician.
- I recommend having or creating a written test with performance review for new staff to ensure their understanding of the treatment and technology.
- W2 employee, rate $15-16 hr with 5% commission on gross sales no matter which team member completes the service. Commission increases up to 10% are considered as raises.
- The typical starting wage for a hospital Registered Nurse (RN) is approximately $16-26; you can recruit an RN right out of nursing school. Some nurses get their license to work in the medical spa industry.

- Offering benefits is optional: If you gain an amazing staff, health benefits will keep them onboard.
- A technician does enter settings and skin response in treatment records.
- A Physician has to initial treatment records for liability and state requirements; this can be done weekly or monthly but must be done.
- Consumables:
- Rolled sheet paper sheet for bed covering
- Water-based ultrasound gel
- Distilled water for the machine
- Disposable or washable hand & larger towels for body covering and gel removal
- Disposable razors
- Tongue depressors
- 70% alcohol and spray bottle – clean up

B.Hifu 4D Monaliza – two handles face and body contouring machine

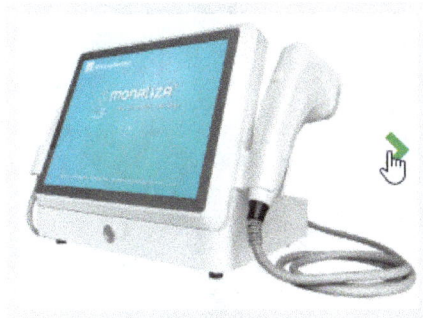

- Benefits of service: this machine provides non-surgical facelifts, melted fat and skin tightening with

no downtime. Clients come in once a month and continue to get results for up to 90 days but can have a second treatment after 30 days. (Most clients come in for one area that bothers them. When that area improves, the other imperfections are more noticeable, and they want to continue with more areas.)

- Two handles, one to get closer to the eye and mouth, the other to get the larger facial and body areas
- Cartridges: 6 for the face, 5 for the body
- Separate Purchase: Roller Cart for machine
- RESULT PHOTOS: My actual clients. Blonde: Two treatments (four areas), Male: three treatments (5 areas), Body one tx (five areas)

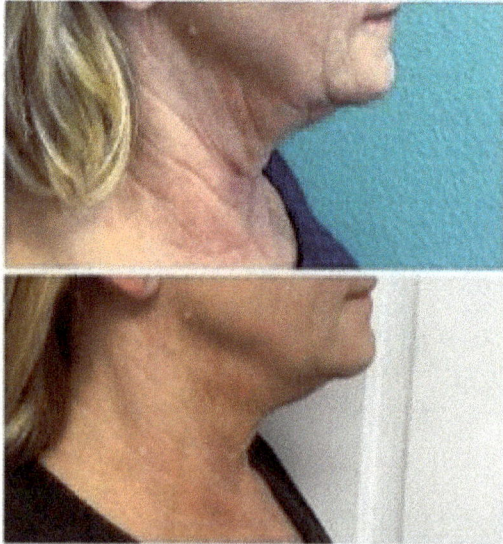

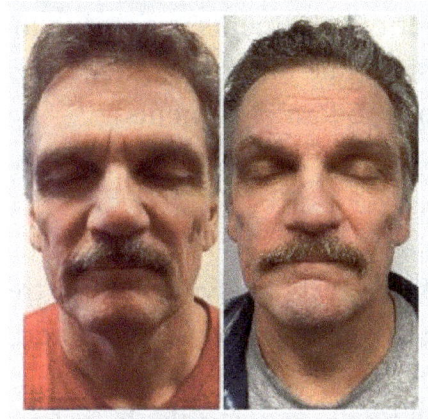

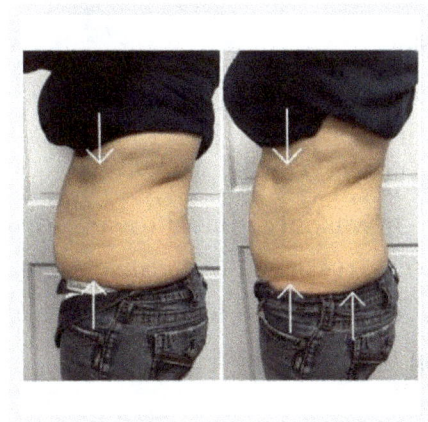

- Target Market:
- Face lifts: anyone over the age of 35
- Body Contouring: anyone over the age of 18
- Pricing and projected income on conservative gross sales for the first year
- Face Lift first-year potential of $36k to $60k
- Body Contouring first-year potential $48k to 84k
- Pricing $250 - $300 an area. The size of an area is approximately 2" x 8" no matter where on the body (packaging multiple treatments I recommend a bare minimum $100 an area)

- The number of treatments varies due to age, health, and volume in the treatment area
- Face lifts: one to four treatments
- Body Contouring: any given area can be 1 to 10 treatments
- Treatment times
- Example: face/neck lifts typically five treatment areas done in one hour, consult and add 30 minutes.
- Staffing will be the same as the laser hair removal machine
- Consumables
- Makeup remover or facial cleanser
- Stretcher sheet or Rolled sheet paper
- Water-based ultrasound gel
- Disposable or washable hand towels for gel removal
- 70% alcohol in a spray bottle or wipe
- Disposable Tissue/cloth to remove makeup and use for cleaning the cartridges

C.Ultrasound & RF – Cellushape & Kumashape

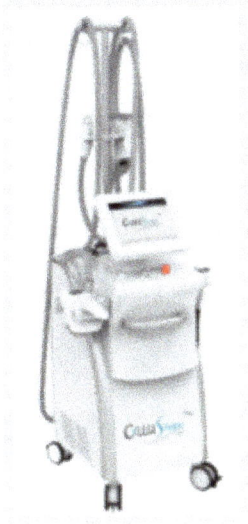

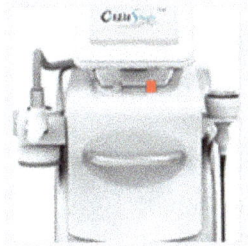

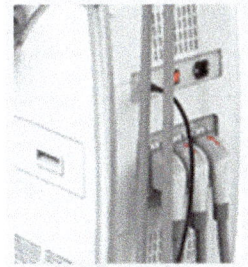

- Benefits of service: Target market kick-starting a weight loss allows for weekly treatments, accountability, and diminishes potential needs for skin removal surgery. There is a large market of people looking for this option, and non-surgical treatments are not marketed this way; this adds to gross sales over a more extended period of time.

- Four handles provide: one ultrasound cavitation, three radio frequency handles that administer RF, infrared light, red light therapy, and vacuum massage.

- RESULT PHOTOS of my actual clients. Far left, stomach, client: she lost 50 lbs. before coming in with lots of loose skin to tighten and some fat to melt. 60-minute sessions once a week for one year, only lost an additional 10lbs in that year, no surgery. Red shirt, stomach, client: six sessions. Male stomach client six sessions

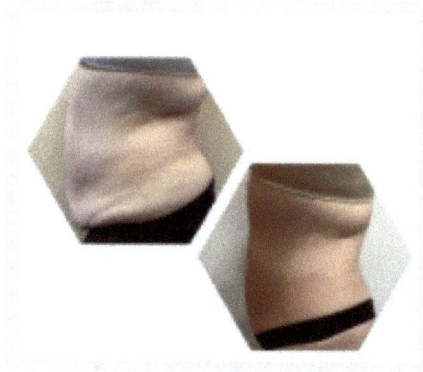

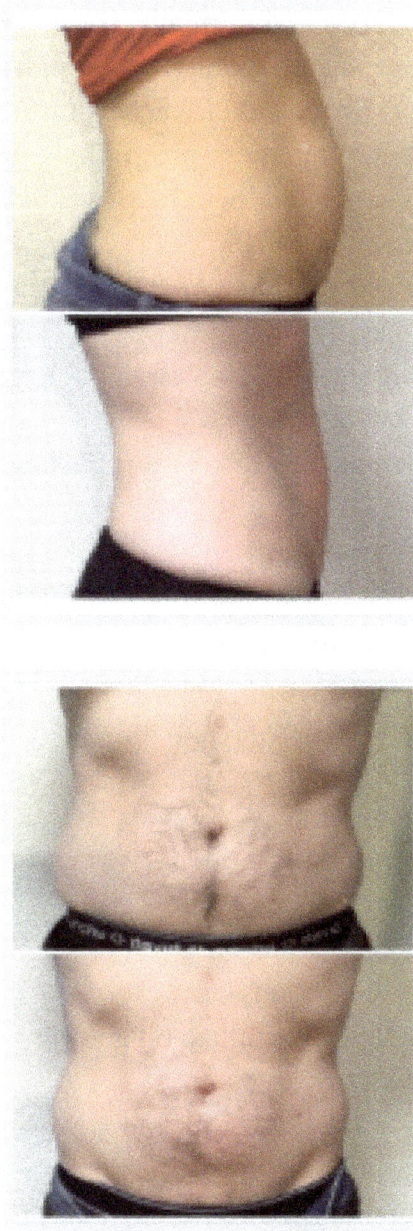

- Target Market, for example, anyone who is interested in major weight loss meal programs. The total client base adds up to $71 Billion in sales in the United States. Additionally, connecting with naturopaths and nutritionists who might see treatments as helping their clients stay on track with their weight management programs.

- Pricing and projected income; projected income in the first year $40k - $70k.
- Pricing is based on time per session, minimum session of forty minutes.
- 40 minutes retail $195, 6 session package discount $149. each = $895
- 60 minutes retail $293, 6 session package discount $225 each = $1350
- The number of treatments a manufacturer recommends is six sessions and get additional results for three weeks with a continued balanced diet and activity.
- Treatment times: (see iii. Pricing and projected income)
- Staffing: Esthetician, W2 starting wage $15, 1099 may charge more per hour
- Consumables
- Grapeseed oil
- Spray dispenser for oils
- Stretcher sheets – minimize oil getting on the treatment bed
- Disposable or washable towel to wipe the client dry after treatment
- 70% alcohol in a spray bottle or wipe

D.Electromagnetic Muscle Trainer

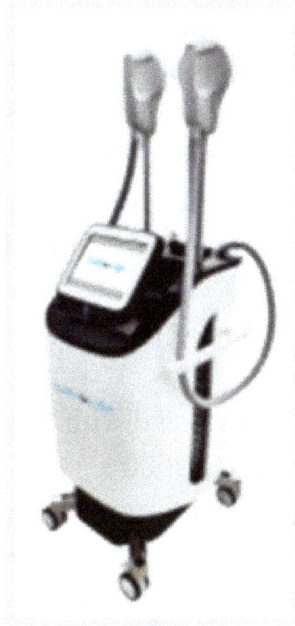

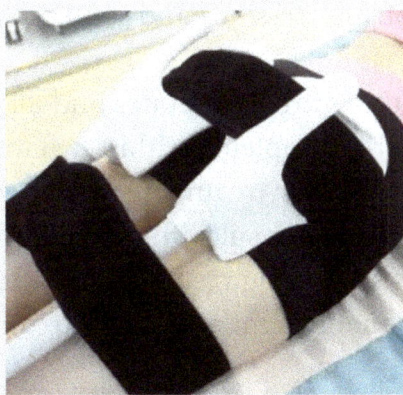

- Benefits of service: Build muscle in less time than going to the gym and can last six months to a year. Building muscle has multiple benefits that include; helping to control body fat, improve energy levels, immune system, and emotional health, reduces stress, builds strength and stamina, helps joint support, promotes bone health and can increase self-confidence. This is a great combination for weight loss clients that can be packaged and alternate with ultrasound/RF treatments.

- This machine can come with two or four handles that with Velcro straps secures to the clients treatment area

- Target Market: Same as the markets listed with the other machines.

- Pricing is usually packaged with four sessions that average $650 each = $2600

- Grand opening special for an example; Buy one session, 1 per person per purchase as a try me special or a $500 package of four sessions $1800.

- The numbers of treatments provided are typically a minimum of four sessions and some up to eight sessions.

- Treatment times are 30 minutes and all four sessions can be completed within two to four weeks.

- Results from all four treatments; (A google search for these treatment results from other providers will show clients still seeing results weeks after the fourth session and clients right after eight treatments.

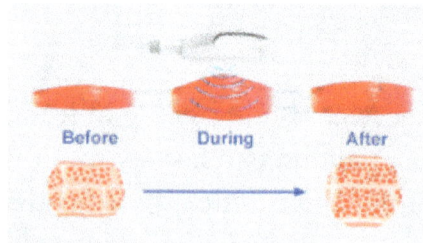

Before   During   After

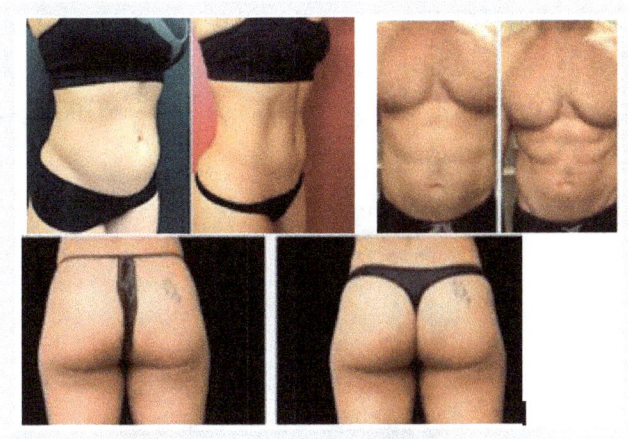

- Staffing: Esthetician, W2 starting wage $15, 1099 may charge more per hour
- Consumables
- Rolled sheet paper or stretcher sheet
- 70% alcohol in a spray bottle or wipe

8. Additional services you can add to your spa and why:

- Rezenerate NanoFacial: Nano-technology allows serums to penetrate deeper into the skin. Improves fine lines, dehydrated skin
- Compliments non-surgical facial treatments, great to add to packages
- Client returns once a month, continues exposure to services and your specials
- This is relaxing, rejuvenating, hydrating, balances the skin tone and exfoliates.
- The machine cost approximately $899, ask for specials and if they have a referral program. www. rezenerate.com

- RESULT PHOTO: My client thought she needed a face lift. After one Rezenerate NanoFacial with the serums, she could see some of the wrinkles were just dehydrated skin.

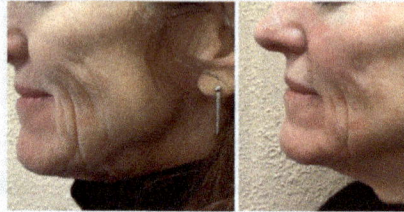

- Staff: Esthetician can be a W2 employee with a possible wage $15, or a 1099 contractor who's wage may be more.
- Pricing: The basic service with me averages $165, adding vitamin C and other hydrating serums averages $200
- Number of Treatments: Rezenerate NanoFacial recommends weekly treatments for four weeks and then once a month.
- Marketing; package in treatments of four
- Profitability; gain returning clients who are exposed to your services and monthly specials. Potential income $ 15k to 30k a year
- Consumables
- Hyaluronic Glide serum. A starter bottle is provided with the purchase of the patented Rezenerate pen; enough for about ten treatments. A larger bottle will treat approx. forty clients and is about $99.

- Individually packaged Nano tips. (With the purchase of the Rezenerate pen you have the option of two different quantities, for example one option is enough for about twenty clients. The variety of tip quantity packs average $ 100-375, example $375 might be fifty tips.
- Facial cleanser.
- Disposable tissue/cloth to remove makeup.
- Recommendation; a hydrating sheet mask for after treatment, ex: MediHeal Collagen Essential Lifting & Firm Mask.
- Retail Products for clients:
- Examples: Hale & Hush has a Vitamin C and Brilliant Eye serum that is a wow-factor finish to the Rezenerate NanoFacial treatment. Please research products to decide what will work best in your spa.
- Procell: Microchanneling is an advanced form of traditional microneedling. Safe for all skin types, long-lasting improvements for a variety of skin issues including: fine lines, wrinkles, acne scars, stretch marks, skin tone, tightening, and surgical scars http://www.procelltherapies.com/referral/angelaj
- Less downtime, as good or better results than microneedling
- Procell has two separate models (Pro and MD), to accommodate your local regulations for estheticians.
- Machine cost: For example, the MD set is approximately $4,000 and can include treatment supplies for up to five or ten clients. All pricing

depends on the current promotion or deal with the
sales representative.

- Ask if a referral program is available.
- Staff: Esthetician, same as Rezenerate
- Pricing: $400 a service. (recommend lowest service
  charge, $300)

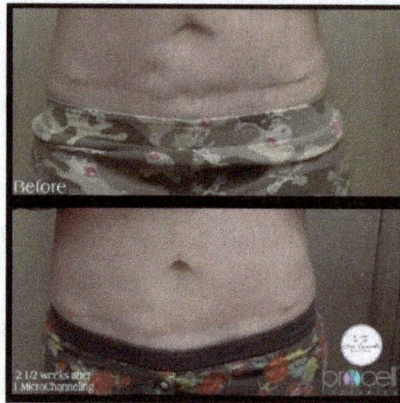

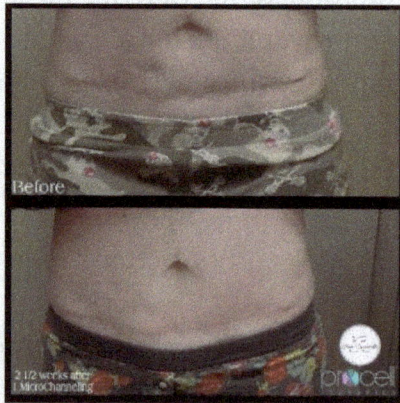

- RESULT photos; please go to the Procell website
  directly. Written results below;

- For deep forehead lines, usually four or more treatments. Deep lines are hard for non-surgical machines to eliminate without penetrating the skin.
- Lines around the mouth and tightening of the neck can be four treatments with the addition of the aftercare kit- it is an up-sale item that does maximize results.
- Scars can see great improvement within three treatments. One kit can be used over three sessions due to the focus on just the scar. You would add-on the cost of a new treatment tip for each session.
- Consumables
- Facial cleanser
- Disposable tissue/cloth to remove makeup
- MD Serum (purchased through Procell only. With the purchase of the Procell machine, depending on the promotion, a five or ten pack of serum is included.
- Face & Body Tips. Purchased through Procell only. With the purchase of the Procell machine, depending on the promotion, a five or ten pack of tips is included.
- Calm & Hydrate Masks-reduces downtime. Purchased through Procell only. Depending on the promotion with your initial purchase a five or ten pack may be included.
- Sunscreen; after treatment if a client has plans afterwards, application of sunscreen is a good idea. I like Tizo3, sample bottles to give to clients. Tip: mention you have a grand opening or major sale promotion starting and the sales representative may

have a good sale, for example a 100 sample bottles for $40.

- OPTIONAL: Aftercare trial kit and Aftercare 30-day care kits, these kits do help maximizing results.

9. Consent forms: Spas have inquired about body contouring consent forms; the manufacturers listed above and Botox/filler providers have consent forms most can provide. Some automatically send the forms, others you have to ask. Overseas manufacturers like Sincoheren are still getting up to speed on the standards for USA Spas. I have a one-page body contouring consent form example in the back of this book. You can copy and edit to fit your state and business requirements. It is always a good idea to consult with an industry business attorney in your state to ensure you have covered all your bases for liability reasons.

A little extra note for those wanting to provide Botox or Fillers; the medical reps can give you consent forms and set your RNs up with master injectors for training. In addition, I have offered three sites in the next paragraph with experienced professional recommendations for RNs wanting more training than what some manufacturer reps may provide, you can check out these websites for more information.

www.merz.com   ,   www.facialesthetics.org   ,   www.twelvetwentyeightwellness.com/

This private Facebook group requires each member to have a specific license to join. The providers are helpful and an excellent way to network in the industry. The group is called "Aesthetic Medicine and Wellness for RNs, PAs, LE"

These are all valuable resources that are above and beyond the training that is received from the Botox/Filler companies.

10. Aesthetic Industry staff expectations:

- Knowledge-driven: wanting to learn about new technology, products, protocol improvements
- Recommend offering some continuing education
- Group meetings to discuss their techniques, researched ideas for potential improved treatment results, confidence, and motivation.
- Constantly striving for client satisfaction – the above will assist
- Desire to experience treatments to best serve clients.
- Working hours: Clarification that expected hours are similar to retail hours.
- Benefits: Most medical spas do not provide benefits. For med spa owners, some basic benefits are recommended to assist in retaining employee's long term.

11. Bonus marketing tips

- Website content: when purchasing off-brand equipment, your web designer should know that adding in key-words in the description that states results are similar to Velashape, Ultherapy, and EmScupt are helpful when potential clients are googling the service.

- Instagram is beneficial in the industry and you need over 100 followers to gain access to analytical and statistical reports. Suggested tips for your Instagram business account;
- Plan to organize your posts by choosing a color theme and font that will be used in each post. This keeps your home page clean, professional, and attractive.
- When you gain access to your reports, you will see peak days and times for when your followers are on line. Assisting in managing your time to schedule your posts on those days.
- Suggested post topics: alternate between inspiration, community support, informational, services you provide, and result photos.
- Hashtags are Important when selecting what ones to use:
- Research local providers with a high count of followers to see what hashtags they are using.
- When deciding on what hashtags to use; stay under the ones with a 300,000 followers count. Please make sure the 15 to 30 hashtags you can use per post include a variety of follower counts, including the low 300 followers (When you use hashtags with higher follower counts it decreases the possibility of followers seeing your posts.)
- Always include your business hashtag in your posts.

12. Summary of Consumables discussed in this book;

- Disposable or washable hand towels (all treatment rooms)
- Disposable or washable body towels (diode laser only)
- Tongue depressors (diode laser, not required but can use with hifu)
- Rolled sheet paper or Stretcher sheets for all treatment rooms
- Water based ultrasound gel (used by diode laser and hifu)
- Distilled water (used by diode laser)
- Grapeseed oil and a spray bottle (used by cellushape)
- 70% alcohol and a spray bottle (all treatment rooms)
- 70% alcohol wipes (Procell)
- MD Serum (Procell)
- Face & Body Tips (Procell)
- Calm & Hydrate Masks (Procell)
- Sunscreen (Procell)
- Hyaluronic glide (Rezenerate)
- Treatment tips (Rezenerate)
- MediHeal Collagen Essential Lifting & Firm Mask (Rezenerate NanoFacial)
- Facial cleanser (hifu, cellushape, Procell, Rezenerate)
- Disposable tissue/cloth to remove makeup (hifu, cellushape, Procell, Rezenerate)
- Your supplier/manufacturer will provide a consumables list for Botox/Fillers

8

PENING A MEDICAL SPA; STAFFING DETAILS, INSURANCE, LICENSING, TREATMENT ROOM AND CONSUMABLES LIST, EQUIPMENT RECOMMENDATIONS

OVER THE YEARS, while participating in multiple Facebook groups there is one question that stands out, "How do I price my services?"

Here is one way to help you price the products used and non-surgical services. I work backwards to ensure that all of my costs have been covered. How this works is to know the three types of costs for your business;

(1) Cost to provide the service (ex. Materials you use plus labor),

(2) Hard expenses (monthly costs that never go away; rent, insurance, administrative duties for overhead), and

(3) Variable expenses (costs that will fluctuate every month, credit card fees, utilities, maintenance, etc.)

The Cost to provide services will vary based on the items used such as; liquid products, solid disposable items, and hourly wages. Each item you use, for example a solid like stretcher sheet, has a cost per case plus shipping and handling. Each item used in your service will need to be broken down to get the cost per service. This will be a bit of work; however, breaking down these costs will be worth your time. Knowing exactly what your service costs and not just pricing the service based on your competitors. The cost per service will help you decide how low you can discount your service or if the service is worth keeping in your spa. *Please know that all the prices used in the proceeding examples are for easy math purposes and will vary based on your true expenses.*

When it comes to Liquids, you can ask your supplier how many estimated treatments you should get out of each bottle. If they do not have this information, I highly recommend performing one service with a measuring spoon. Yes, your liquid back bar containers are labeled in ounces. This is an easy conversion using google. As an example, your treatment uses one teaspoon of liquid product. You can google "how many teaspoons in an ounce," the result will show six teaspoons. If the liquid product contains three ounces you will take six multiplied by three giving you 18 treatments. (6 teaspoons x 3 ounces = 18 treatments.) As a provider you may know that the amount of product used may fluctuate between clients so I typically lower the calculation down to seventeen in case I use more product on a client versus another. To find the cost per service, if the three ounce bottle cost you $40 divide that by 18 treatments equals **$2.22 a treatment**.

For Solids, such as gloves, cleansing wipes, paper bed covering or bed stretcher sheets, paper towels, and tissues.

Each of these items is sold in a boxed quantity. An example for a breakdown on stretcher sheets, sold in a boxed quantity of fifty the price averages $31 for the case plus shipping $9 total solid item cost, $40.00 (31+9=40.) To find your cost per service, you already know you will only use one stretcher sheet per client, so you will take the total cost and divide it by the quantity which in this case would **equals eighty cents a treatment**. ($40\50= .80)

The final cost to breakdown is the service provider's hourly wage. You will need to decide if you will pay yourself or someone else an employee a wage (W2) or an independent contractor fee (1099).

Real quick, the simplified difference between W2 and 1099; a W2 is an employee you pay a wage, report and pay the taxes you withhold and with the hours you set for them they can, with proper training, assist with administrative tasks, clean up tasks, laundry, front desk, provide services, and you would provide all supplies necessary for them to complete these tasks. Make sure when you hire the employee, they understand the positions related tasks they are expected to attend to within the working hours you assign. The wages you pay this employee, for the cost per service calculation I typically double the wage to ensure I cover the federal, state and local taxes. For example, you pay the employee $15 an hour, for cost per service you would **use $30 in the calculation**.

A 1099 an independent contractor will agree to a set wage for the duties you both have agreed upon for the work to be performed. The independent contractor will report or invoice you for their hours worked and you would pay them. At the end of the year you will file a 1099 with the IRS and mail a copy to the independent contractor. They will pay their own federal, state and local taxes. Be sure to consult your accountant or CPA for more specifics on what is required from you. For the breakdown per service you would **use the agreed upon wage for the calculation.**

Now, if you are a solo entrepreneur and you want to bring home $35 an hour, I double the wage per hour to cover the taxes. You have the options as you grow to decide with your accountant if you will pay your taxes quarterly or at year end. As a solo entrepreneur **the hourly wage would be $70.**

Should you decide to hire someone to provide administrative duties only, the same concept applies and would be considered in the hard expenses that do not change. If you are solo and want $35 an hour (doubled is $70), the average administrative tasks take 15 minutes per service hour performed. Seventy divided by four equals $17.50 per service hour). Total labor for one service hour with administrative duties as a solo provider would be $70 plus $17.50 equals $87.50. **With an employee providing the service and administrative tasks it is $30 plus $7.50 equals $37.50.**

If you are just starting your business and not sure what you want to make an hour, here is one my consultant provided. Start with knowing how much you want to make a year. For the sake of this example we will use the, national average, Estheticians gross salary $50,000 working 40 hours in 6 days a week. This is based on the hours and days I worked while becoming an esthetician, mostly evenings and Saturdays. Now that we have these numbers we will break it down to determine the hourly wage; $50,000 divided by twelve months equals $4,166 a month. Now divide $4,166 by four weeks in a month, equals $1,041.50 a week. Knowing the weekly gross total of $1,041.50 divided that by forty hours and this works out to $26.04 an hour. So doubling the wage to cover taxes is $52.08 per service. (For calculation of cost per service for hard expenses make note that forty hours a week times four weeks equals 160 hours a month.)

Hard expenses, for example total $945 a month would include items such as;

- rent/lease $500
- phone/internet $100
- all insurance costs $80 (professional, general, property, workman's comp)
- booking software subscription $40
- membership subscriptions $25
- Short term hard expenses might be;
- A loan payment for your treatment machines $200 (unless you leased the machine and then it would be an ongoing hard expense.
- Business startup loan or after covid an SBA disaster loan

The cost per service breakdown for hard expenses would be to take $945 divided by 160 working hours a month equals **$5.91** per treatment hour.

Variable expenses for example total $300 and would be items such as:

- Miscellaneous office supplies $50; even if you don't think you need them every month it is good to have it in the equation.
- Marketing expenses, like Facebook ads) $150
- Professional fees $100 (accountant)
- Utilities typically are your rent/lease; if the electric/gas is not included your utility company can provide the monthly average.

For the cost per service of variable expenses you would divide $300 by 160 working hours **equals $1.88 per treatment hour.**

Here is a thorough example of the "Cost per service" breakdown for laser hair removal. For easy math purposes I will use the hard and variable expenses from the details we just reviewed. The list of supplies for this service includes;

- Stretcher sheet **$1 per client**. The breakdown; one box has 25 stretcher sheets at $25 (price includes taxes and shipping)
- Ultrasound gel **$1.25 per client**; a 5 liter container (with taxes and S/H $25) that fills twenty 10oz bottles. $25 divided by 20 bottles equals $1.25 (for the sake of this book say 1 bottle used per client)
- Razor **32 cents** (if client did not shave). A pack of 100 razors is $32 (with taxes & S/H). Take 32 divided by 100 equals 32 cents.

- Towel laundry labor, **$8.99 per client**. I recommend towels to clean up the gel after a treatment versus paper towels. The breakdown for the towel laundry includes the cost of laundry detergent, dryer sheets and labor. Apply the same concept breaking down the cost per load of laundry as you did with the bed sheets, ultrasound gel and razors.
- For the labor, timing myself I know it takes 5 minutes to load the towels into the washer, 5 minutes to put them in the dryer, 5 minutes to unload the dryer and 15 minutes to fold the towels equaling 30 minutes for laundry. If you have to take the towels home to wash, add in the time to commute to and from where you wash the towels. My travel time was 30 minutes round trip, making laundry labor one full hour.
- Laser hair removal machine payment per treatment **$5.00**. Not knowing how much I would use the machine, I went with how many hours I want to use the machine on treatments a month; I chose 40 hours a month. My loan payment is $200 a month; $200 divided by 40 hours equals $5 per treatment.
- Treatment Labor **$37.50**; for this example I chose a forty-five minute treatment session for a large area, this includes an employee technician plus the administrative person and taxes $ 37.50. This is the amount from our labor breakdown from earlier. When you want to know what your minimum cost per treatment area is, even if it only takes 15 minutes, remember the administrative time is still about 15 minutes to any service.

- Add in hard expenses **$5.91**
- Add in variable expenses **$1.88**

After breaking down the six components to provide a laser hair removal treatment I added the bold amounts to bring the total cost per service with a 45 minute treatment and 15 minute administrative tasks **equals $61.85**, the breakdown; **$1 + $1.25+ $.32+ $8.99+ $5+ $37.50 + $5.91 + $1.88 equals $ 61.85**. You need to remember this is your actual costs and does not include profit. To ensure you make a profit most businesses will mark up the actual costs up to fifty percent for their products, consumables and labor. For example the new calculation would be **$2+ $2.50+ $.64+ $17.98**+ $5 **$75**+ $5.91 +$1.88 equals $110.91

If you have provided laser hair removal treatments you know that some of the treatments can take as little as fifteen minutes with the client, however the administrative tasks are still fifteen minutes. The only part of the calculation that would change is the employee technician wages; $30 divided by four, equals $7.50 and add $7.50 for fifteen minutes of administrative work, equals $15.00 for wages instead of $37.50. I personally do not break it down this far because I choose to work in one hour calculations. Please remember the amounts used in these calculations are not real numbers. They will vary depending on your specific equipment choices, rent, insurance and consumables that you purchase. As you move forward in your business you will eventually pay off loans that affect your cost per treatment. Do not deduct that cost out of your total cost per treatment. At some point in the future there may be repair charges or equipment replacement costs and this will allow you to have reserve funds to cover those costs.

The value of knowing what it costs you to do business per service is priceless. Especially in helping you determine what kind of specials you can run in comparison to your competitors.

Wrapping up this chapter on how to price your services I want to share how to research your competitors. When I am consulting with other medical spas I will google my client's competitors within a 60 mile radius from their location. If their pricing is not on their website you can always call and state you are checking local providers for this service and want to know what their specials are for the month or regular price for the service. When you are checking out your competitors make sure they are using the same technologies, they don't have to be the exact same machines. Also make note if you and your competitor are using a name brand machine versus a technology comparable machine, also called off-brand machine. A lot of times the service price will be lower when the provider uses an off-brand machine for the same service. One other good search is to check the national average cost of the service you are providing. Here is an example of Coolsculpting versus Coolplas. The technology is the same, the machine costs are very different and so you will see pricing for Coolsculpting average about $800 a treatment area and Coolplas average is $400 a treatment area.

As I close this chapter I would like to remind you about the workbook questions included, it is a good tool to help retain the details provided. If you have any questions, please email me at contournetics@gmail.com. If the questions are simple I am happy to answer at no cost. Should they become more involved, I may recommend scheduling a consultation to have a full discussion over the phone or via a Zoom meeting. My goal is to help you optimize your business, boost gross sales, retain happy clients who love raving about you, and refer your services.

WORKBOOK QUESTIONS

BELOW ARE questions designed to help you retain key details that were provided in this book.

What is the purpose of fat cells?

What are toxins?

How do toxins leave the body?

What are the two types of fat cells, and where are they located?

When exercising, which of the two types of fat cells burns and leaves the body first?

How does the lymphatic system get activated?

When the lymphatic system is flushing toxins, what levels in the body does it affect?

Why do clients see results on the same day?

What layers of the skin does non-surgical contouring affect?

How do you tell the difference between loose skin and fat volume?

What are the 5 factors that affect a client's body shape and size?

How long should you be active each day?

Which activity is preferred after a non-surgical contouring treatment, cardio or weight lifting?

When building muscle, what does the body focus on more?

What is the value of water intake?

What are the causes discussed that cause hormone imbalance?

What happens to the skin after the age of 35 or childbirth?

In general, how many types of technology are being used in the non-surgical contouring industry?

Does cryolipolysis provide skin tightening?

With cryolipolysis, what is the crucial post-care task needed right after treatment?

How often can you receive cryolipolysis treatments?

If the treatment area hardens after a cryolipolysis treatment, it is called?

What is the benefit of cryotherapy?

Why would laser lipolysis have a cooling system in the applicator?

When receiving laser lipolysis, how often can you have a treatment?

How far away is the radio frequency applicator designed to keep away from directly touching the skin?

Is radio frequency best for melting fat or tightening skin?

How far does infrared energy heat penetrate the skin?

Why is red light therapy combined with infrared?

What is the top benefit of electromagnetic therapy?

Where can you apply electromagnetic therapy treatments on the body?

How long can the results last after electromagnetic therapy?

At what range in hertz would ultrasound be effective in melting fat?

Does ultrasound go through the skin, tissue, and then to the fat cells like the other technologies?

How does the ultrasound applicator handle work on the body?

How does the applicator handle differ between the broad ultrasound and the intensified ultrasound?

What is the treatment area size for intensified ultrasound?

What happens to the fat cell with non-surgical contouring versus surgical lipo?

Who provides you with the list of treatment contradictions?

What is key, during a consultation, and why is it important?

What is a red flag you should keep in mind?

When assessing a treatment area like the belly overhang, what is another element that helps you determine how to get your client optimal results?

What should you do before touching a client, and why is it important?

When assessing how many treatments a client needs, what is something they need if they have more than 2 inches to eliminate?

Define the three types of clients? (Fine-tuning, budging stubborn areas, and weight loss journey)

What were the recommended technologies for the weight loss journey type of client?

How is keeping your vehicle oil changed similar to non-surgical contouring?

What effect can a quality conversation have on clients at each visit?

Why are taking result photos important?

What are the two details you should look for with your camera?

Why would you want a designated area and clear client placement tape on the floor?

What are the recommended outside resources you could have available to clients?

Why are outside resources valuable?

How can you stand out from your competition if you already have a client base?

If you are in a small or large city, what is one element of marketing that is great for both?

How would you market to those starting a weight loss journey?

Benefits of gaining the trust of your community?

What is the benefit of knowing the different belly shapes, and what they might indicate?

What are stretch marks similar to, and how do we treat them?

If a client does not want a tummy tuck after childbirth, what can you recommend a new mom do to minimize, if not eliminate, the need for one?

After surgical liposuction what treatment can you provide?

How many types of Cellulite are there, and which is the hardest to eliminate?

How many factors affecting Cellulite did we discuss, and what are they?

How is cooking an entire meal in one skillet and cleaning it related to non-surgical contouring?

What are the stages of lymphatic obstructions?

Can you eliminate Cellulite permanently, and why?

GLOSSARY

1099
A 1099 form is an information return that reports taxable income other than wages, salary, and tips. A 1099 independent contractor uses their own methods and sets their own schedule. The payer of these services will file a 1099 form that goes to the IRS and a copy to the service provider. The service provider includes the 1099 income reported when they file their other taxes at the end of the year and is responsible for the federal and state taxes on that amount.

https://www.entrepreneur.com/money-finance/what-is-a-1099-form-everything-you-need-to-know/442401

https://www.entrepreneur.com/growing-a-business/w-2-or-1099-why-it-pays-to-classify-your-employees/246139

Aesthetics
of, relating to, or dealing with <u>aesthetics</u> or the beautiful

Blood Pathogen Clean Up Kit
Spill clean-up supplies including Red-Z Fluid control solidi-fier, biohazard scoop, disposable towel and biohazard bag. https://www.redcross.org/store/bloodborne-pathogen-personal-protection-kit/711216.html

Botox
to inject <u>botulinum toxin</u> into (part of the body and espe-cially part of the face) especially for cosmetic purposes (as to minimize wrinkles)

Botulism
acute food poisoning that is caused by <u>botulinum toxin</u> produced in food by a bacterial <u>clostridium</u> (*Clostridium botulinum*) and is characterized by muscle weakness and paralysis, disturbances of vision, swallowing, and speech, and a high mortality rate

Broad Ultrasound
Is a term I personally use to help clients understand and differentiate between the standard ultrasound cavitation wave that is used in the larger cylinder shaped handles, because the wave is not constricted and discharges out of the handle in a cone shape into the treatment area; versus the focused intensified ultrasound wave used in the HIFU and Ultherapy machines as discussed in this book

Candida

any of a genus (*Candida*) of parasitic fungi that resemble yeasts, occur especially in the mouth, vagina, and intestinal tract where they are usually benign but can become pathogenic, and have been grouped with the imperfect fungi but are now often placed with the ascomycetes

Cellulite

deposits of subcutaneous fat within fibrous connective tissue (as in the thighs, hips, and buttocks) that give a puckered and dimpled appearance to the skin surface.
The clinical classification of cellulite proposed in 1978 by Nürnberger & Muller graded this condition in 3 levels of severity: mild, moderate, and severe. https://www.ncbi.nlm.nih.gov/pmc/articles/PMC9298294/

The European aesthetic industry appears to have generated names for the three different grades of cellulite that has taken off in the U.S. aesthetic industry. No one source has been located for the individual who generated these terms.

Chakras

any of several points of physical or spiritual energy in the human body according to yoga philosophy

Cholesterol

a steroid alcohol $C_{27}H_{45}OH$ that is present in animal cells and body fluids, regulates membrane fluidity, and functions as a precursor molecule in various metabolic pathways and as a constituent of LDL may cause atherosclerosis

Circulatory System

the system of blood, blood vessels, lymphatics, and heart concerned with the circulation of the blood and lymph

Collagen

the system of blood, blood vessels, lymphatics, and heart concerned with the circulation of the blood and lymph

Connective Tissue

a tissue of mesodermal origin that consists of various cells (such as fibroblasts and macrophages) and interlacing protein fibers (as of collagen) embedded in a chiefly carbohydrate ground substance, that supports, ensheathes, and binds together other tissues, and that includes loose and dense forms (such as adipose tissue, tendons, ligaments, and aponeuroses) and specialized forms (such as cartilage and bone)

Contouring

an outline especially of a curving or irregular figure

Cortisol

a glucocorticoid $C_{21}H_{30}O_5$ produced by the adrenal <u>cortex</u> upon stimulation by ACTH that mediates various metabolic processes (such as gluconeogenesis), has anti-inflammatory and immunosuppressive properties, and whose levels in the blood may become elevated in response to physical or psychological stress

CPA
Certified public accountant is an accountant who has met the requirements of a state law and has been granted a certificate

Cryotherapy
the therapeutic use of cold

Dermis
the vascular, thick layer of the skin lying below the epidermis and above the superficial fascia that contains fibroblasts, macrophages, mast cells, B cells, and sensory nerve endings and has an extracellular matrix composed of proteoglycans and glycoproteins embedded with collagen and elastin fibers also known as the Dermal Layer

Dunlap
An Urban Dictionary word to discribe when someone's belly "dunlapped" over their belt or waistline. www.urbandictionary.com

EIN
An **Employer Identification Number** (EIN) is also known as a Federal Tax Identification Number, and is used to identify a business entity. www.irs.gov

Elastin
a protein that is similar to collagen and is the chief constituent of elastic fibers

Electromagnetic Muscle Stimulation

high-intensity focused electromagnetic energy. For example; A single EMSCULPT session feels like thousands of powerful muscle contractions which are extremely important in improving the tone and strength of your muscles.These powerful induced muscle contractions not achievable through voluntary contractions. The muscle tissue is forced to adapt to such extreme condition. It responds with a deep remodeling of its inner structure that results in muscle building and sculpting your body.*
https://bodybybtl.com/solutions/emsculpt/

Epidermis

the outer epithelial layer of the external integument of the animal body that is derived from the embryonic epiblast

Esthetician

a person licensed to provide cosmetic skin care treatments and services (such as facials, hair removal, and makeup application)

FDA

Food and Drug Administration (FDA) is responsible for protecting the public health by assuring the safety, efficacy, and security of human and veterinary drugs, biological products, medical devices, our nation's food supply, cosmetics, and products that emit radiation. The FDA also provides accurate, science-based health information to the public.
https://www.usa.gov/federal-agencies/food-and-drug-administration

Fluidity

the physical property of a substance that enables it to flow

Glycation

a spontaneous non-enzymatic reaction of free reducing sugars with free amino groups of proteins, DNA, and lipids that forms Amadori products. The Amadori products undergo a variety of irreversible dehydration and rearrangement reactions that lead to the formation of advanced glycation end products (AGEs) https://www.ncbi. nlm.nih.gov/pmc/articles/PMC5643203/
Also a buzz word in the beauty industry to summarize AGEs (Advanced glycation products) https://www.skininc.com/ science/physiology/article/21884163/glycation-and-the-skin

Gross Sales

Gross sales, also called top line sales, are the total of all product and service sales reported by an organization during a period not including any returns, discounts, or rebates. https://www.myaccountingcourse.com/accounting-dictio nary/gross-sales

Hertz

 a unit of frequency equal to one cycle per second

HIFU

Abbreviation for High Intense Focused Ultrasound machine, the same technology as Ultherapy brand name machine.

HIPAA

Abbreviation for Health Insurance Portability and Accountability Act of 1996; a federal law that requires the creation of national standards to protect sensitive patient health information from being disclosed.
https://www.cdc.gov/phlp/publications/topic/hipaa.html

Hormone Imbalance

A hormonal imbalance happens when you have too much or too little of one or more hormones — your body's chemical messengers. It's a broad term that can represent many different hormone-related conditions.
https://my.clevelandclinic.org/health/diseases/22673-hormonal-imbalance#:

Hyaluronic Glide Serum

One of the highest concentration Hyaluronic Acids that can be found on the market today! Great to use as your infusion serum and/or slip serum for the Rezenerate portion of your NanoFacial.

This clinical strength Hyaluronic Acid (HA) formulation holds up to 1000 times its weight in water. As a component of skin tissue, HA boosts the skin's moisture content exponentially, reduces inflammation, triggers cell-communicating abilities, and reduces moisture loss.
https://rezenerate.com/product/hy-rez-glide/

Hydraulic Massage Table

A hydraulic massage table comes with hydraulic lift actuators that help you easily adjust its height to ensure the most comfortable experience for both client and masseuse. Hydraulic stationary massage table models can be manual or electric. Manual lift systems with crank handles are more affordable, while electric ones with foot control are more convenient.
https://www.massagewarehouse.com/shop-by-department/massage-equipment/stationary-tables/stationary-tables/

Hypodermis

the tissue immediately beneath the epidermis of a plant especially when modified to serve as a supporting and protecting layer

Independent contractor

Independent contractors work for themselves; the companies they work with don't technically employ them. It's essential for employers to correctly classify independent contractors to comply with the U.S. Department of Labor and the IRS.

Independent contractors submit invoices for their work and are subject to self-employment tax. The paying company doesn't deduct tax from their payments.

https://www.businessnewsdaily.com/15853-independent-contractor-employee-differences.html

Jowls
usually slack flesh (such as a dewlap, wattle, or the pendulous part of a double chin) associated with the cheeks, lower jaw, or throat

LE
Abbreviation for Licensed Esthetician

Liposuction
surgical removal of local fat deposits (as in the thighs) especially for cosmetic purposes

Lymph Fluid
a collection of the extra fluid that drains from cells and tissues (that is not reabsorbed into the capillaries) plus other substances. The other substances include proteins, minerals, fats, nutrients, damaged cells, cancer cells and foreign invaders (bacteria, viruses, etc). Lymph also transports infection-fighting white blood cells (lymphocytes).

https://my.clevelandclinic.org/health/articles/21199-lymphatic-system

Lymphatic Blockages
a blockage of the lymph vessels that drain fluid from tissues throughout the body and allow immune cells to travel where they are needed. https://medlineplus.gov/ency/article/001117.htm

Lymphatic system

the part of the circulatory system that is concerned especially with scavenging fluids and proteins which have escaped from cells and tissues and returning them to the blood, with the phagocytic removal of cellular debris and foreign material, and with the immune response and that consists especially of lymphoid tissue, lymph, and lymph-transporting vessels

Microneedling

a form of therapy that utlilizes instruments containing rows of thin needles that penetrate the dermis to a uniform depth, creating a controlled skin injury. This controlled skin injury induces rapidly-healing micropunctures with subsequent stimulation of collagen and elastin fiber production, resulting in skin remodeling. https://www.ncbi.nlm.nih.gov/books/NBK459344/

Mommy Pouch

Fat stored below the waist line on Women who have given birth to several children. https://www.urbandictionary.com

PA

Abbreviation for Physicians Assistant

Paradoxical Adipose Hyperplasia

a rare, previously unreported side effect of cryolipolysis with an incidence of 0.0051%. a delayed increase in adipose tissue at the treatment site.

https://www.ncbi.nlm.nih.gov/pmc/articles/PMC4171727/

PCOS
polycystic ovary syndrome

Photobiomodulation
A form of light therapy that utilizes non-ionizing forms of light sources, including lasers, LEDs, and broadband light, in the visible and infrared spectrum

https://www.ncbi.nlm.nih.gov/pmc/articles/ PMC4390214/

Reiki
a system of touching with the hands based on the belief that such touching by an experienced practitioner produces beneficial effects by strengthening and normalizing certain vital energy fields held to exist within the body

RN
Abbreviation for Registered Nurse

SMAS Layer
The superficial musculoaponeurotic system, or SMAS, is often described as an organized fibrous network composed of the platysma muscle, parotid fascia, and fibromuscular layer covering the cheek. This system divides the deep and superficial adipose tissue of the face and has region-specific morphology. https://www.ncbi.nlm.nih.gov/books/ NBK519014

Stretch Marks

indented streaks that appear on the abdomen, breasts, hips, buttocks or other places on the body.
https://www.mayoclinic.org/diseases-conditions/stretch-marks/symptoms-causes/syc-20351139#:

Triglycerides

a system of touching with the hands based on the belief that such touching by an experienced practitioner produces beneficial effects by strengthening and normalizing certain vital energy fields held to exist within the body

Ultrasound Cavitation

use of ultrasound technology to break down fat cells below the skin. This procedure involves applying pressure on fat cells through ultrasonic vibrations. The pressure is high enough to make the fat cells break down into a liquid form.
https://www.webmd.com/beauty/what-to-know-about-ultrasonic-cavitation

Ultrasound Wave

A wave of frequency above the audible frequencies the human ear. In medical diagnostics are used ultrasound frequencies between 3 and 10 MHz
https://www.ncbi.nlm.nih.gov/pmc/articles/PMC3564184/

W2

A form used by employers to report wages, salary and taxes that the employer has withheld and paid directly to the federal, state, local and city tax offices for the employee. An employee is generally subject to the company's instructions about when and where to do the work; what tools or equipment to use; and what order or sequence of tasks to follow. If the employer has the right to control how the work results are achieved, or the employee must be trained to perform services in a particular manner https://www.entrepreneur.com/growing-a-business/w-2-or-1099-why-it-pays-to-classify-your-employees/246139

https://www.irs.gov/forms-pubs/about-form-w-2

9

GENERIC FACE/BODY CONSENT FORM

I UNDERSTAND that the Face and Body Contouring device used during the procedure uses high frequency intensified ultrasound and/or broad ultrasound, with the option to use radio frequency, micro current and that results may vary client to client. I understand that there is a possibility of short-term effects such as reddening, blistering, scabbing, temporary bruising, temporary discoloration of the skin, severe headache or nausea and that these have been fully explained to me.

Results may vary depending on individual factors including medical history, skin type, patient compliance with pre/post treatment instructions and individual responses to treatments. I understand that this nonsurgical treatment may involve more than one treatment and the fee structure has been fully explained to me and because of the individual nature of the treatment we cannot offer refunds but will make every effort to insure the best possible results and outcome for our clients.

I certify that I have been fully informed of the nature and purpose of the procedure and expected outcomes and possible complications and I understand that no guarantee can be given as the final result obtained. I am fully aware that my condition is of cosmetic concern and that the decision to proceed is based solely on my expressed desire to do so.

I confirm that: (Please put a check mark by each item listed below that is true and accurate to your understanding)

____ I am not pregnant at this time

____ I do not have a pace-maker, other electronic or metal implants

____ I do not have a heart transplant, disorder or disease.

____ I do not have Acute Inflammation and do not take anti-inflammatory medications daily.

____ I do not have High Blood Pressure and/or has been under steady medication for over 6 months.

____ I do not have a Neurological disorder.

____ I do not have High levels of Triglycerides (hereditary).

____ I do not have a serious infectious disease.

____ I do not have severe or active cystic acne or open wounds/lesions in the treatment area

____ I do not have any medical condition that could have any adverse effect from this treatment.

I consent to the taking of photographs and authorize their anonymous use for the purpose of tracking program results, research, education and promotion.

I certify that I have been given the opportunity to ask questions and that I have read and fully understand the contents of this consent form.

Client Signature _____

Date_____

Client Print Name _____

GET YOUR QUESTIONS ANSWERED

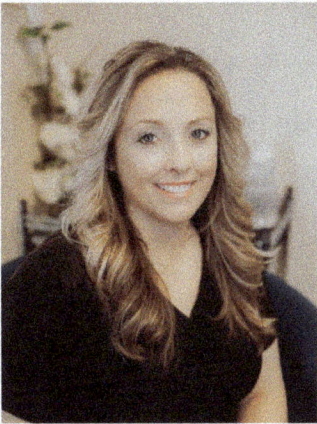

I'VE BEEN in your shoes; providing services, asking questions, not getting answers I needed and feeling like something was missing.

Marketing issues...

While living in a rural manufacturing city with consumers burnt out from gimmicks, I successfully built and sold my spa business.

Started all over in a new State. In a hospitality town, lots of money and cautious consumers who only purchased services based on word of mouth. My business survived 2020 and still thriving.

My passion is nonsurgical body contouring

I have been the client who turned into a passion driven service provider, trainer and consultant.

The industry has boomed so quickly that states, schools, and manufacturers are striving to keep up.

When that happens... Information gaps happen

I listened to clients, participated in multiple groups to listen to providers, added their questions to my experience and dove deep into researching the answers. Additionally being a national certified trainer for a manufacturer gave me insight into the technologies to help providers.

One Hour: Coaching/Consultation

Get answers to your nonsurgical contouring questions.

Book Your One Hour Consultation: https://cavi-cinch.square.site/

Book Your One Hour Consultation/Coaching Session:

Visit https://cavicinch.com/contournetics

Purchase the 80 minute Video Seminar for Staff Training:

www.ingramcontent.com/pod-product-compliance
Lightning Source LLC
Chambersburg PA
CBHW060233030426
42335CB00014B/1438